NUTRITION
FOR A
BETTER
LIFE

Peter Brabeck-Letmathe is Chairman of the Board of Directors at Nestlé S.A. He started his career at Nestlé in 1968 as salesman and product manager for icecream. From 1970 to 1987 he worked for Nestlé in Chile, Ecuador and Venezuela, later transferring to Nestlé's international headquarters in Vevey, Switzerland, where he took on worlwide responsibility for Culinary Products. In 1992 he was appointed Executive Vice President of Nestlé S.A. with worldwide leadership of strategic business groups while simultaneously being in charge of Marketing Consumer and Corporate Communications, and Public Affairs. In 1997 he was elected as a member of the Board of Directors and appointed Chief Executive Officer of Nestlé S.A., a position from which he resigned in 2008. Since 2005 he has been Chairman of the Board of Directors at Nestlé S.A. Peter Brabeck-Letmathe also serves as Vice Chairman of the Foundation Board of the World Economic Forum in Davos and board member of several companies.

Peter Brabeck-Letmathe

NUTRITION FOR A BETTER LIFE

A Journey from the Origins of
Industrial Food Production
to Nutrigenomics

Translated from German
by Ian Copestake

Campus Verlag
Frankfurt/New York

The original edition was published in 2016 by Campus Verlag with the title *Ernährung für ein besseres Leben. Eine Reise von den Anfängen der industriellen Nahrungsproduktion zur Nutrigenomik.* All rights reserved.

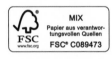

ISBN 978-3-593-50597-8 Print
ISBN 978-3-593-43437-7 E-Book (PDF)
ISBN 978-3-593-43457-5 E-Book (EPUB)

Cover design: total italic, Thierry Wijnberg, Amsterdam/Berlin
Editorial assistance: Ruth E. and Friedhelm Schwarz
Typesetting: Marion Gräf-Jordan, Heusenstamm
Printing: Beltz Bad Langensalza GmbH
Printed in Germany

www.campus.de

CONTENTS

Chapter 8:

FOREWORD
Prof. Dr. Patrick Aebischer

Less than twenty years ago, the UN Committee on Economic, Social and Cultural Rights (CESCR) defined the right to food. It is the "right of every individual alone or in community with others, to have physical and economic access at all times to sufficient, adequate and culturally acceptable food that is produced and consumed sustainably, preserving access to food for future generations". Availability, accessibility, adequacy and sustainability: a rather ambitious definition. And just when we, humans, define the right to food, scientists (notably the then chief UK scientist J. Beddington) predict that by 2030, the demand for food will increase by 50%, for energy by 50%, and for water by 30%, thus creating a *'perfect storm'* of global events. Today (2015) 793 million people still go hungry—down from 927 in 2007. We will need innovation, policy, and behavioral changes to fight this storm. Science and technology, universities and businesses must make a significant contribution.

Can the world population of 2030—that's 8.5 billion people—be fed equitably, healthily and sustainably? The good news is that hunger in its most extreme form has decreased globally from over 1 billion in 1990–1992, representing 18.9 percent of the world's population, to 842 million in 2011–2013, or 12 percent of the population. To meet future food demand, agricultural productivity must increase everywhere, particularly among poor farmers. Meeting this challenge requires continued innovation in food processing and packaging to deliver safe, nutritious, and affordable food. It requires reduction of waste and losses, improved crops tolerant to stress, pollution by smarter use of water, fertilizers and new pesticides. We must do it all. The question is not whether productivity should be raised to address hunger and malnutrition. The question is how to achieve this. Increasing yields alone will not suffice.

We need a "greener" Green Revolution. The first Green Revolution technological package had a hefty environmental load. Now, a new vista focused on resilience and sustainability, and also wellbeing, is replacing—or adding to—the productivist paradigm. Solving this new equation requires integrative science, appropriate technology, farmers' knowledge and participation, a performing industry and informed consumers.

Today the world produces enough food for all to go without hunger. Yet hungry many are. On one hand, the source of hunger, is poverty: hungry families do not have the means to buy food. On the other, the culprit is the food system: today, one-third of produced food is eaten by pests or rots away. We need to make agriculture more efficient.

Medicine is moving towards the "4Ps", becoming a predictive, personalized, preventive, participatory medicine. Should farming not benefit from the same approach? Smart farming that integrates local knowledge, cutting edge science, appropriate technology, big data, farmers, smartphones, and businesses. Precision farming that leads to better yields through genotype improvement, exact fertilizer input, proper nutrient ratios, adequate irrigation schedules, geospatial techniques of soil identification, and appropriate mitigation of pests and diseases. Precision farming has the potential to reduce the use of external inputs and thus maximize resource efficiency.

Different forms of farming can and must coexist, our current awe for local organic farming notwithstanding. Strengthening local food systems needs appropriate investments in infrastructure, packaging and processing facilities, and distribution channels, keeping in mind that two out of three humans will live in cities by 2050. Two important strands of agriculture–genetic engineering and organic farming–will also have to be judiciously incorporated to help feed the growing population in an ecologically balanced manner.

Former UN secretary general Kofi Annan pledges to use digital technology to clear away one obstacle to progress for the hundreds of millions of African smallholder farmers: their profound isolation. Africa's smallholders are more than capable of feeding the continent if they are able to use the best agronomic practices. "Most have not adopted these improvements, however, because they don't know about them," says Kofi Annan; "using digital technology to reach smallholder farmers to help them organize holds out the potential for another agricultural revolution." The first Green Revolution increased productivity; the 'Green Data Revolution' will create a smarter, more flexible and resilient food system.

Precision farming incorporates appropriate knowledge and practices, and the green data revolution: this marriage of high tech and local improvements is one key to success. As a small, telling example, consider the initiative run by Nespresso and the non-profit organization Technoserve in South Sudan. The program enables farmers to set up cooperatives, raise funds, invest in infrastructure, and commercialize their coffee for export. It combines local *savoir-faire* and top notch technology. In less that two years, it facilitated the creation of three coffee exporting cooperatives in the south of the country, the first commercial coffee to leave South Sudan in over 30 years.

Food security and empowerment of farmers through science is one part of the story. Olivier de Schutter, the special rapporteur to the UN on the right to food, reminds us that the narrative of nutrition changed in a fundamental way when the UN launched its new Sustainable Development Goals in 2015. It moved from a sole focus on undernutrition alleviation and food security to one that includes food quality, equity and food systems, with a central focus on *malnutrition* in all its forms. Malnutrition is indeed a critical public health problem. It affects the most vulnerable populations: children, the elderly and the sick; individuals afflicted with disease, injuries, in social isolation or with limited resources. Malnutrition affects an estimated 30% to 50% of hospitalized adult patients in the United

States. According to the WHO, in 2012, two billion people lacked essential vitamins and minerals.

Are science and industry tuned to answer the challenge of malnutrition? One science-based response to malnutrition is nutrigenomics, the application of genomics tools in nutrition research to understand better how nutrition influences metabolic pathways, how "diet-regulated" genes are likely to play a role in chronic diseases, how nutrients affect people differently. Ultimately, nutrigenomics will lead to efficient dietary-intervention strategies. Industry plays a crucial role in delivering these individualized or group-specific products to the customer.

Nutrient needs should be met primarily by the quality of food. Food science and engineering do produce—or intend to produce—healthier foods. Yet processed foods are increasingly seen as problematic. We do not realize that almost all foods currently consumed are processed. The three pillars of our Greek ancestors–olive oil, wine, and bread–are all processed. We tend to forget the benefits of the modern food system: lower food losses, better preservation and availability, improved nutritional status, convenience and choice. To get the best nutrition, to fight malnutrition, we need all the tools we can get. Fortunately, food engineering is benefitting from the rapid convergence of nanotechnology, biotechnology, computer science and cognitive sciences, opening fascinating new avenues. These include food structuring, package engineering, digestive system simulation and modeling, understanding the bio-availability of nutrients, the mechanisms of satiety and the role of genetic predispositions.

Food engineering is also driven by a number of major food companies. Large company research centers have created an environment in which food research is cutting edge. Food science is one field where universities and industry need each other. Research in nutrition seems pointless if we cannot deliver it to customers and patients; it requires highly qualified human resources and expensive equipment, typically located at universities. Moreover, food science creates plenty of qualified jobs. Indeed, the best food science should embrace universities, industry, *and* the art of cooking—chefs—, because food is more than just its components.

Nutrition engineering can boast many successes, the "super broccoli", oligosaccharide prebiotics and Lactobacillus acidophilus probiotics in yogurt, whole grain–rich foods, low-gluten foods, foods without allergens and smaller portion packages. Despite this, nutrition engineering is often viewed as "nutritionism", the simplistic reduction of food to its nutrient components, and unfavorably compared to "whole foods". While mishaps litter the history of processed food—such as low-saturated, high-trans fatty acid cooking oils—the global attack on processed food is unwarranted. As chef Anthony Warner says, "Food is not good for you based on where it was produced. Nutritional value depends on what the food consists of. ... Natural does not necessarily mean healthy, processed does not necessarily mean unhealthy. We should love fresh food and cooking from scratch, but we should love facts even more. If we, scientists, politicians, health professionals, journalists and chefs continue to distance ourselves from all convenience food, we will distance ourselves from real, time-poor consumers and never change a thing".

I commend Peter Brabeck for a timely book. It is a time of increasing challenges to food system resilience, of the indispensable juncture of the health and sustainability agendas, on the verge of a data-enabled revolution in agriculture. His unique insights are a valued contribution to this most important challenge of our century, feeding nine or ten billion people equitably, healthily and sustainably.

INTRODUCTION

The greatest human desire has always been to lead a healthy and long life. To date, we have already brought this goal a lot closer. Since the mid-19th century, the health of broad social groups in the US and in Europe has improved significantly. The average life expectancy of newborns doubled in both Britain and Germany from 41 and 37 years respectively in 1871 to 80 years in 2015, while in Japan this has now increased from 37 to 85 years.[1] Worldwide, life expectancy in 1820 was 26 years[2] and in 2013 it was 71 years[3].

This development is a crucial part of the result of ever improving nutrition. Only industrial production of food and logistics have provided a sufficient amount of inexpensive, nutritious high quality and risk free food for the broad mass of populations in the cities and the countryside. Medicine has also made parallel advances in the fight against infectious diseases and in the area of hygiene that can be compared with those in food production.

Meanwhile, not only in the US and in Europe, but also in many other parts of the world an affluent society has emerged. By 1996, a clear relationship between the amount of available calories and increasing life expectancy could be detected in highly industrialized societies. The number of calories available has since risen further, but the life expectancy curve has leveled off.[4]

In the last decades, the quantitative growth in food production has not brought people in Western affluent societies any additional benefits. Diseases of affluence such as cardiovascular disease, diabetes and obesity have reached epidemic proportions, and the risk of developing Alzheimer's disease increases with each year that we get older. For food manufacturers, this means refocusing and generating knowledge of products with new properties, which reach far beyond the replacement and reduction of sugar, salt and fat in food.

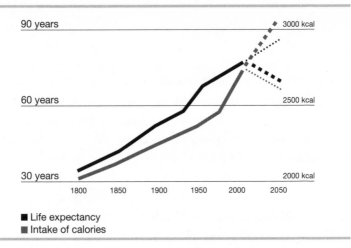

Fig. 1: Correlation between life expectancy and intake of calories

Even in ancient times people were aware that there is a relationship between diet and health. For centuries this realization was the most important foundation of medicine. Medical knowledge was based almost exclusively on observation. Because simply too little was known about the functioning of the body, false and ineffective treatments and recommendations were the rule rather than the exception. To date, there are doctrines that promise a long and healthy life, without being able to provide reliable evidence for their accuracy.

In fact, due to the progress in the various fields of research in the life sciences, the relationship between diet and health has been put in a completely new light. If we change our habits in a similar manner, we can already optimize our health sustainably and prevent certain diseases. The potential is still far from exhausted.

Therefore, the issue of health in the coming decades will trigger a wave of innovation in the food industry. Its advanced technology will play a crucial role in improving the health of entire population groups. The role of science-based personalized health nutrition in the future is to find efficient and cost effective ways to prevent and treat the acute and chronic diseases of the 21st century.

The key messages of the book are summarized in six theses that follow this introduction.

The first chapter begins with the consumers and the question of which diet trends will determine the future, what trends we had in the past and how they were intertwined with the general social developments and changes. This is followed by a consideration of changes in food production, taking account of consumer needs, environmental considerations and resource conservation. The third part of the first chapter offers a first look at the new sciences, which are gathered under the umbrella of the Life Sciences.

The concept of industrial production has been linked positively to many everyday products such as cars or computers. Even products from the entertainment industry are highly appreciated. Compared to this, the food industry has found it more difficult to be perceived positively in today's society.

In the second chapter, I therefore want to take a mental journey through time to show the contribution of the food industry to the progress of humanity, and show the potential future challenges for this industry.

The third chapter will take stock of the present situation of world food, by focusing on overall social development and change.

Food research is discussed in chapter four. Their findings gain much attention in the media and among the public. But many researchers are content to confirm already existing findings and recommendations. Others enter into a competition with their scientific colleagues and try to outdo or disprove them through the publication of ever more shocking reports. At the end the consumer is left completely unsure by the flood of information alone. Therefore, I turn in the fifth chapter to the responsibility of the food industry, while in the sixth and seventh chapters I deal with the responsibilities of policy makers and the individual. Chapter eight provides an outlook on future developments.

In this book, I attempt to look into the future. Not in the form of speculative science fiction, but on the basis of what is being researched today. The research results will be available in a few years and could revolutionize food production to the extent that we come closer to the realization of the human dream of a healthy and long life. We should not miss this opportunity.

For those who want to learn more about the background and other areas of my ideas and actions, I recommend they read my biography (Friedhelm Schwarz: *Peter Brabeck-Letmathe and Nestlé–a portrait. Creating value together*, Bern of 2010). Information on the WHO guidelines on the subject of sugar, salt and fat can also be found in the appendix.

Peter Brabeck-Letmathe
Vevey/Schweiz, September 2016

THE FUTURE OF FOOD—PERSONALIZED, SCIENCE-BASED, RESOURCES EFFICIENT, CARING

1. The challenge

We all desire a long and healthy life. This requires in the future basic dietary changes: a healthy diet for a growing world population can only be ensured if new scientific knowledge becomes part of the production of foods, if the lifestyle of people is oriented toward the goal of a healthy, long life and with a food system efficiently using natural resources.

2. The model

There will not be a uniform approach to healthy eating for everyone, but rather a personalized diet for different population groups. These differences may be either of a genetic or epigenetic nature, based, for example, on age or dependent on the specific life situation.

3. The responsibility of science

The Life Sciences will provide knowledge on a completely new basis with regard to the relationships of biological functions in the human body, nutrition and health.

4. The responsibility of the Food Industry

On the basis of the scientific knowledge of the life sciences, the food industry is developing products and services for a personalized diet for different populations. It provides these services to preserve resources and be socially beneficial for the greatest possible number of people.

5. The responsibility of politics

Social systems and health systems have to be changed from the treatment of existing diseases to the precautionary prevention of diseases. An open market must enable an efficient allocation of resources and comprehensive innovations.

6. The responsibility of each individual

People need to aspire to a new holistic quality in their personal lifestyle and diet and be supported by educational institutions, the media, the producers and processors of food and the food trade.

CHAPTER 1:
ON THE WAY TO NUTRITION OF
THE FUTURE

The reasons why we will feed ourselves differently in the future, is due to the results of scientific research, the manufacture of food and of course constantly changing consumer behavior. Worldwide, consumers will change their behavior and habits in the next 20 years much faster than was the case in the past 60 years. This is due to growing wealth and knowledge and the fact that we are already have technical possibilities in food production that were unthinkable a few decades ago.

However, increasing prosperity not only brings improvements but, as experience shows, even problems. It is not only the companies that have to face the challenges of globalization, it is also every individual who must adapt to global changes and while this is indeed experienced mostly as an advantage it can sometimes be a disadvantage.

Industrial manufacturers of food products are on the one hand expected to supply the ever-growing world population, while on the other hand they have to satisfy the consumption needs of increasingly differentiated consumer groups. 60 years ago, the challenge for the food industry was mainly to produce more and better. Today they must additionally meet an extensive list of demands in terms of sustainability, resource conservation and environmental considerations. They not only do this because of a call by consumers and the politics behind them, but because they have also learned themselves to recognize that growth today in terms of security for the future depends on recognizing new conditions as it was in the first decades after the Second World War.

In the sciences in the 1980s new fields of research began to be opened up. Today we are at the point of implementing that research to put this new knowledge into practice and so give people what they want most, namely health and a long life.

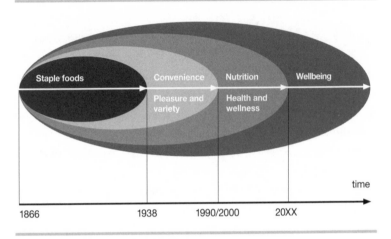

Fig. 2: The next Step: extensive wellbeing

Global megatrends on the consumer side

"Panta rhei–everything flows", this saying from the Greek philosopher Heraclitus could also be the guiding principle for the field of trend research. Our world is in a constant state of flux, something which is not perceived by most people, because they are part of it themselves. The changes and developments in the depths of the global society are like currents in the ocean, which develop into a large force.

Megatrends change the world slowly, but for the long term and fundamentally. If a new Apple iPhone hits the market, which is perhaps a trendy product, it does not constitute a trend or a megatrend. Mobile communication, which began in the early 1990s, however, is an excellent example of a megatrend, as it has changed the lives of most people fundamentally. Trend researcher John Naisbitt saw it already in 1982,[1] before either mobile phones or the internet were available to the general population. Ten years later, in 1993, there were 34 million mobile phone connections, and by 2015 there were 7.085 billion worldwide. On Earth, there are therefore almost as many mobile phones as people (7.3 billion).[2]

Food trends that describe how our diet will look like in the future will be determined by a number of megatrends. Conversely, changes in eating habits for the trend researchers are also indicators that permit conclusions to be made about the emergence of new megatrends. For the future development of nutrition the following megatrends are of particular importance:

- an increasingly aging society,
- the increase of chronic diseases and
- an ever growing health consciousness, which is based largely on the first two trends.

There are also other strong factors that will influence our eating habits in the future. This also means that more and more people are living in ever larger cities, which must be supplied with food, and marks the emergence of a new lifestyle due to the demands and opportunities of globalization, which is described as a trend regarding the 'individualisation of life'. This also has a far-reaching influence on what we eat, when we eat and where we eat.

1 out of 5 will be older than 65
70 % of developed countries will have more 50+ than 50- In China more than 200 mio. will be older than 65 • Healthcare systems will have to cater to the needs of older people

3 out of 5 will die of a chronic disease
50 mio. Alzheimer patients 7 % of adults worldwide will suffer from diabetes • Increased prevention and treatment of chronic diseases

1 out of 5 will be overweight or obese
120 mio. in the USA 20 % of all minors in China • Necessity to treat concomitant diseases (coronary diseases, diabetes)

Worldwide healthcare spending will be up to 5 to 10 trillion Dollars
More than 16 % of the GDP will be spent on healthcare In the USA healthcare expenditure will reach 14.000$ per capita • Costs will have to be kept in check and/or funding will have to be increased

Fig. 3: Global health ecosystem—by 2020

The Silver Society—On the road to an aging world

On every continent more people reach a higher age than ever before. This applies to industrialized countries, the emerging economies and the least developed countries, although at different rates depending on the starting position of the respective societies. The rapid growth of aging populations is not only a challenge to social systems, but also to food manufacturers, because every age, from babies to the very elderly, needs a diet that is tailored to their very specific situation and based on current knowledge.

The year 2050 is expected to see a world population of 9.7 billion people.[3] The number of over-60s, which is now around 841 million worldwide, is expected to grow to over two billion by 2050. Of these 360 million will be older than 80 years and three million older than 100 years. 2020 will be the first time in human history that more people are aged over 60 in the world than children under five.[4] The reason we are getting older is primarily due to increasing global prosperity, which ensures better nutrition and medical care. Currently there are two billion people worldwide on the way out of extreme poverty and moving towards a life that offers sufficient material supplies.[5]

The fastest current increases in life expectancy are of people in Latin America and Asia. In Latin America, an average age of at least 70 years is predicted for children who were born in 2012. In Asia, life expectancy between countries is still very different. Top place is occupied by the residents of Singapore and Hong Kong, and it is quite possible that they will catch up with the levels found in Western industrial countries, or even outstrip them. Today, however, Europe is still in front.[6]

After Japan, Italy and Switzerland, Germany is the country with the fourth highest average age of population. In 2030, more than half of the people will be over 50 years old in Europe. The further life expectancy of 50-year-olds will then be another 40 years. One assumes that by 2030 in industrialized countries more than a third of the population will be 65 years and older. At the same time the proportion of people in Asia over 60 will be already more than half of the population.[7] In the US, 37 percent will be more than 50 years old and a good 20 percent over 65.[8]

Demographic change leads to a general change in society. Not only will lifestyles and consumption change due to the growing population of older people, but also the requirements of social and healthcare systems. The older ones will want to maintain in their subsequent years the lifestyle that they have acquired in the 30 years before the age of 60. In the US, the majority of the population feels old when they reach 80 years. In Germany, this feeling is, on average, already felt at 77 years. But if one looks at the average life expectancy in these countries, then the difference in the period in which people feel old is only three to five years. The perceived age of the people in these countries is between ten to 20 years lower than their actual biological age.[9]

So today people have a completely different self-perception. This is a reason that the young and middle-aged people compare their lifestyle and their way of life with that of the very old. Many people reach old age with hardly impaired health. The expectation of being able to spend one's life in health, the so-called "healthy life expectancy," is always improving because medicine is able to treat acute diseases, accidents, as well as infections better and delay the onset of chronic illness. In addition, more and more old people come to believe that they can postpone the aging process and its symptoms through their personal behavior.

The feeling of old people as being really old, is mitigated by urbanization and increasing mobility. Currently this produces a "Multi-aging culture"[10] with many individual forms of aging. More and more old people because of their life experience are concerned about cohesion in a changing society. Health and nutrition concepts do not have for the elderly an orientation in their past, as is commonly expected. But the willingness to shape the process of aging itself is now far greater in the elderly than it was in previous generations. This attitude carries over to the offspring.

In many developed countries, the elderly are the only growing consumer group, because the current 50 plus consumer generation is accustomed to its purchasing power, is mobile and familiar with modern communication media.[11] The classic "first health market", consisting of doctors, hospitals, health insurance, nursing, pharmaceutical and biotechnology companies as well as medical technology, becomes more and more reliant on the older "second health market" which includes alternative medicine, coaching, wellness and sports facilities, as well as nutritional counselling and the entire food industry.[12]

What the elderly need is a diet that promotes wellbeing and makes them feel good. However, this food is not to be presented as for "seniors" or as "baby food for pensioners," but the challenge to the food industry, is to provide a differentiated food supply that meets the metabolic demands of aging people and in taste and presentation is no different from what younger people are used to eating.

Chronically ill people are defined as those treated for at least one year for the same disease at least once a quarter by a physician. In Germany, in 2010 two out of five people met this definition.[13] In the US, chronic diseases (including cancer) are responsible each year for seven out of ten deaths, causing 86 percent of total national health care costs.[14] One of the main problems is the metabolic syndrome, a complex system of morbid obesity, causing disturbances in lipid metabolism, type 2 diabetes and cardiovascular disease. According to the International Diabetes Federation (IDF) in 2014 387 million people worldwide suffer from diabetes.[15] Two thirds of them live in developing countries. By 2035, the IDF predicts an increase in world diabetes patients to 592 million.

More than a billion people from a total of 6.7 billion in 2008 are overweight, or around 15 percent. By 2050 this will apply to about 20 percent of the estimated 9.6 billion population, say the United Nations.[16] In the US, more than 170 million people who are aged 18 or older, are overweight (2014), while it is not just adults who suffer from this. In China, 20 per cent of under-18s will be overweight and the percentage of overweight male minors in Brazil, Mexico and Russia is already higher than in Germany.

Professor Ganten, the organizer of the Berlin World Health Summit, stated in 2010 that we export the so-called lifestyle diseases to poorer countries. That there are more and more chronically ill is caused among other things by the fact that we are living longer and so the number of risk factors increases. Diabetes is a typical disease of aging, as is dementia. Today, there are 55 million patients with dementia and by 2050 their number will have nearly tripled to 135 million.[17]

The majority of chronic diseases such as cardiovascular disease, diabetes, obesity, cancer and respiratory diseases can be attributed to a relatively small number of risk factors. These include smoking and excessive alcohol consumption, obesity, high cholesterol and hypertension. "We eat too much and eat poorly. We are moving too little. To get chronic diseases of the cardiovascular system and obesity under control, for example, we need in the first place to change the diet, "said Professor Ganten.

It is therefore important that from kindergarten we eat healthily, consuming a less salt and sugar-rich diet and so develop an understanding of what our bodies need.

"There is much talk about cost, but I believe that the real challenge is educational. This is the best sort of vaccination, and a basic requirement for healthy behavior, "said Ganten, the former head of Charité in Berlin. "We will never achieve a society that is completely free from disease. This a part of life, "said Ganten. "But we need to avoid the mistakes we make in many areas".[18]

Worldwide approximately 57 million people died in 2008, 36 million of them to non-communicable diseases. 17 million deaths were due to cardiovascular disease, 7.6 million to cancer, 4.2 million to chronic respiratory diseases and 1.3 million to diabetes. These four groups of diseases are thus responsible for about 80 percent of deaths from non-communicable diseases. Being sedentary alone accounts for 3.2 million deaths.[19]

Anyone who thinks such civilization diseases mainly affect people in industrialized countries is mistaken. On every continent except Africa the number of deaths due to chronic diseases now exceeds the number of deaths caused by infectious diseases.[20]

To combat the global health problems of the world population successfully, requires the cooperation of all stakeholders that deal with people's diets. It will not be enough in the future to appeal only to people's reason and their own responsibility. The consumer must participate in combating health problems themselves but, for various reasons, this is often not happening. Also to rely on the medical care of people by physicians and pharmaceutical manufacturers given the size of the problem does not offer a satisfactory solution.

Therefore, in particular, the food industry and the retail and hospitality sectors are required. We all rely, from the producer of fast-food to the consumer, on the manufacture, sale and consumption of complete food groups such as meat and sausage products, non-alcoholic soft drinks, confectionery and certain baked goods. But consumers above all are not ready to change because food is also about enjoying life.

The health systems of all countries will need support from the food industry, as the cost of health care associated with non-communicable as well as chronic diseases continue to rise. After all, as professor Ganten states, already 70 to 80 percent of health care costs, are accounted for by non-communicable diseases (especially dementia, cancer and diabetes).

The trend towards growing health awareness

When is one actually healthy? Professor Ganten has an answer: "What health is can be difficult to sum up. And certainly to measure. Because if you look hard enough, you will find in each body a few time bombs. Also one must not add requirements to the concept of health which overwhelm the individual." If you can do what others expect from you and you from yourself, then in their eyes you are pretty healthy.[21] Health is therefore a question of self-perception, and the difference is whether one feels sick when one is sick.

Modern health consciousness has its roots in the period after the Second World War, when it was found that the hitherto biggest killers such as pneumonia, tuberculosis and gastrointestinal disease had been replaced by cardiovascular disease and cancer. The United States Public Health Service (PHS) wanted to find out why coronary artery disease (CAD) was the leading cause of death in the US and what risk factors led to heart attacks or strokes. Therefore in 1948 a systematic study began of the population in the town of Framingham in Massachusetts. Known as the Framingham Heart Study, the investigation initially covered a period of 20 years. In the initial phase, around 5,200 men and women between 30 and 60 were selected who at that time had no cardiovascular disease. In 1971 the children of the study participants were then involved, so that inter-generational observation was possible. Into the 1990s, the study was then continued, and it is still one of the most important epidemiological studies in the United States.[22]

Overall, the known risk factors were identified here. During the investigation, it turned out that life-threatening symptoms could be at least reduced by a change of lifestyle by each person concerned. The recommendation was the reduction of obesity, control salt intake, take antihypertensive agents, exercise and, of course, end smoking. So in this study you could find the basis for the idea that preventive measures promote health sustainably.

In addition, the Framingham Heart Study showed that a modern lifestyle and plentiful consumption did health more harm than good. Numerous subsequent studies have examined these results and confirmed them.

The role of health in today's competitive society

Above all, the consumers of the so-called Millennial Generation are interested in new trends, and health related to the ingredients in their food. They often prefer artisanal and natural products that are GMO or gluten-free or are organically grown. Due to their busy lifestyle they want fast solutions, consumer ready-made portions and clear information. Fixed meals are less and less the norm and snacks are becoming increasingly popular. One reason is changing family structures. In many societies, the number of single-parent and single-person households is growing and millennials are increasingly asking for a diet with additional health benefits. They will live a longer, more active and healthier life in all probability.

In December 2012 the *Social Trends Health* study by Tomorrow Focus Media examined what people do in today's competitive society to stay healthy and fit. 91.2 percent of respondents consider health the most important thing and are very interested in it. The majority of young people have a keen interest in health. For the under 16 year olds, this is already at 74.3 percent and for the over-55s reached a value of 96.7 per cent.[23]

86 percent also pay attention in everyday life to their health and 67 percent forego their love of things like alcohol, cigarettes or sweets. Diet and exercise are the factors that have the highest priority in order to stay healthy. Nearly half of all respondents also seek information on health from the internet. This is not surprising, because the search engine Google provides 180 million entries for the search world "health". Around 20 percent of those interested in health topics get their information from the print media which today covers almost all health issues.

Especially for the large audience that it is opposed to treating health issues pragmatically it is necessary to create additional psychological incentives (nudging) about health claims to encourage more people to take care of their own health. The entire field of "e-Health" will be part of the second health market that will play an increasingly important role. Smartphones and tablets serve as mobile devices not only for communication but also for the measurement of vital signs. This goes from the recommendation of certain foods on supermarket shelves to calculating the nutritional needs of the customer beforehand.

Already every 23rd app worldwide is a Health App.[24] In the two major app stores iTunes and Google Play, in early 2015 there were around 80,000 apps in the categories medicine and health and fitness. The number of Android Health Apps was more than 30,000. In addition, there are about 46,000 health iOS apps. Here lies the opportunity to make the connection between personal measurement and control systems or digital fitness tools and sources of Big Data. Today the audience of LOHAS (Lifestyles of Health and Sustainability) makes use of these services. But similar to the use of smart phones it is to be expected that these offers from e-Health will develop from status symbols to self-evident devices and applications for use in everyday life by broad sections of the population.

The trend towards "being-one's-self", to perceive oneself confidently, to distinguish yourself from others, without becoming isolated and not be lost amid the masses is particularly evident in the field of nutrition. To meet the individual consumer's highly differentiated needs, a highly fragmented supply of foodstuffs has emerged in supermarkets, something that makes it easier for the consumer while often making it difficult for them to orientate themselves.

Individuality is understood as freedom of choice, how to make one's life, and particularly the details, part of a whole. This includes what you eat how, where and with whom.

What we eat is always the possibility for self-realization, self-experience and not least for self-expression. Food creates identity and is regarded by many people as an expression of their beliefs. All this is of course only for those who live in affluent societies, or at least enough have food, and of course not for those who go hungry.

Today we live in a time of "Consumer Confusion", because there is a lot of negative news related to food preparation and lots of information that contradicts each other. The consumer is missing the advice amid the recommendations and offers that gives him or her the ability to choose the appropriate healthy diet. It is clearly the task of the food industry, in cooperation with public authorities (health authorities, schools, etc.) and the scientific community to provide help by making it clear and transparent which foods are good or less good for a person's health.[25]

Through innovation and the improving of products, Nestlé ensures that they contribute to healthy diets and are responsive to changing consumer demands. In the United States, for example, it was early in offering such specialized products as Lean Cuisine, while establishing itself as a brand that catered for the modern diet. The new range of Stouffer's Fit Kitchen with at least 25 grams of protein per serving, complex carbohydrates and vegetables is primarily aimed at male consumers who according to research miss good, nutritious meals from frozen products.

Most consumers when choosing their diet move between the two poles of a sense of security by custom on the one side and the wish to try something new, on the other. Humans are evolutionarily and as such set out to constantly look for what is new. Whoever is among the first to try something new has an experience advantage over others and thereby revaluates himself on this basis. So it is not surprising that even with food there is always something new to be tried.

Globalization and urbanization support this trend. More than half the world's population now lives in cities. In 2050 there nearly 70 percent of the world population according to United Nations projections will live in cities. Quality of life there depends on many factors and one of them is that the food supply corresponds in price and quality to the needs and possibilities of city dwellers.[26]

The tasks of the new food science

In April 2005, at the initiative of the International Union of Nutritional Sciences (IUNS) and the World Health Policy Forum, an international workshop was held in Giessen, whose aim was to develop a new comprehensive definition of nutritional science. Renowned scientists from around the world, dealing in various disciplines with dietary issues, participated in this workshop. The result was adopted in the Declaration Giessen (Giessen Declaration) and presented in September 2005 at the 18th International Congress of Nutrition (ICN) in Durban.[27]

The definition of the new Nutrition (Nutrition Science) reads as follows:

"The food science deals with food systems, food and drink, the nutrients contained therein, and other ingredients as well as their interaction in and between all relevant biological, social and ecological systems.

The task of food science is to contribute to a world in which present and future generations can exploit their opportunities to live in good health and to develop, preserve and enjoy an increasingly diverse environment.

Nutritional science should be the basis for food and nutrition policy. This in turn should mean the identification, creation, preservation and protection of rational sustainable and equitable regional, national and global food systems allow to secure the health, welfare and the integrity of mankind and also the biological and physical world."[28]

This statement is, of course, far beyond what constitutes classical nutrition science in its focus on the development of new products and production processes. It is questionable whether the classical food industry and traditional food science are able to accept such newly formulated challenges or effectively implement them.

Equally questionable is whether the pharmaceutical industry and their research institutions would be willing and able to use its resources and instruments to solve the health problems of billions of people. We at Nestlé have thoroughly examined to what extent cooperation between pharmaceutical companies, drug development and food companies and food research is possible and discovered that the structures of the two sides are not strongly compatible with each other, since the food industry is primarily consumer oriented while the pharmaceutical side focuses on searching and marketing new drugs. So what we need is a new integrative scientific perspective, which is also able to provide a new industry with research results that can be passed as actual products or services to the consumer.

We therefore set up a new company called Nestlé Health Science as the relevant scientific counterpart of the Nestlé Institute of Health Sciences. There are two main aspects, the study of the basics of health and then converting this knowledge to improve health, prevent disease or cure.

Life Sciences—A new dimension of science as a solution

The field of Life Sciences, also called biological science or *Lebenswissenschaft* in German, includes all those research branches of science and engineering that deal with processes and structures of living organisms. These not only include human and animals but also plants and microorganisms. The life sciences include numerous branches of biology, such as agricultural research, biotechnology, human biology, cell biology, genetics, molecular biology and neurobiology, as well as medicine, biomedical research, biochemistry, biophysics, bioinformatics, genomics and nutritional science and food research.

Progress in various disciplines of the life sciences have enabled the emergence of a strong food research field, the aim of which is to develop food that keeps us healthy and prevents diseases or finds cures.

The fact that a relationship exists between diet and people's health has been known since antiquity. However, scientific explanations in support were slow to be established. Only in the middle of the 19th century were chemists able to identify the major components of a diet, which included proteins, carbohydrates, fats and water. At this time, food was regarded almost exclusively as an energy source, with quality measured on the basis of the number of calories. That changed in the early 20th century with the discovery of vitamins and other micronutrients, which, despite not providing energy, were found to be necessary for the body's metabolism.[29]

In addition to vitamins, among the micronutrients that the human body must absorb are minerals and trace elements, which were discovered when scientists examined the association between malnutrition and diseases such as scurvy. In 1911, vitamin A was discovered, followed a year later by vitamin B and at the beginning of the 1920s vitamin C. After 1930, these vitamins were successfully and inexpensively synthesized.[30]

At the time, nutrition research was at the forefront of the development of health. There were numerous studies conducted among the population, which enabled general dietary recommendations to be derived from their findings. But often this proved fruitless because, as we know today, people are very different in both their genetic and metabolic systems.

Because of advances in genetic research, especially since the complete decoding of the human genome in 2001, and the study of the genomes of many of our food crops, nutritional science has now been able to examine dietary components at the molecular level. As a result the new research field of nutrigenomics emerged, which examines the interactions between our diet and our genes.

Nutrition researchers try to figure out why certain foods are healthy for some of us yet less healthy for others. Thus the basis for the individual processing of food is our very own personal metabolism, and how well this works. The effect of all substances that we eat depends on their conversion and degradation or storage in the body. Here, the individual embodiments of the metabolic components, for example the enzymes, are determined to a large extent by our individuel genomes. Depending on the enzyme version that one has, one human's metabolism can work more or less efficiently than another person's.[31]

A well-known example that shows that there is indeed a link between genes and diet is the fact that most Asians do not have a good tolerance for alcohol and can feel its effects after the first beer. Around half of them have a less efficient form of the enzyme whose job is to break down alcohol in the liver. When a person does have a less efficient form of the enzyme then naturally the body can not clear the ethanol as rapidly as another with a genetically more efficient form of the enzyme. However, conversely the Japanese can digest raw fish much better than Europeans.

Our cells do not always use all their available genes. Throughout our life, and depending on specific circumstances, we only switch on a selection of our genes (expression), while the rest remain off. This principle is called gene regulation. There are many ways in which genes can be turned on or off. Sometimes there are long-term effects of gene regulation caused by age, environment, lifestyle or disease.

Nutrition researchers have examined dietary components with regard to their influence on the regulation of gene activity. In doing so they found certain food components which after the digestion process are able to penetrate the interior of cells and act like a switch to turn certain genes on or off. This is especially true for genes that are important for metabolism.[32]

For those looking for correlations between diet and genetics huge amounts of data have to be processed, which is now possible thanks to current advancements in technology and bioinformatics. So nutrition researchers gladly take advantage of the enormous capacity of investigative genomic tools, leading to the development of so-called gene chips such as those designed to examine single nucleoide changes in the human genome. With their help a person can be analyzed for millions of gene variants at once and reactions to nutrition, such as body weight, cholesterol, medical history, can be measured or requested directly from the individual. When searching, for example, for whether associations between certain genotypes and nutrition responses can be found, then the more people you can examine the better.

One thing is relatively certain: There is no specific form of nutrition which is best for everyone, such as the often-touted Mediterranean diet, based on the mere consumption of olive oil and plenty of fruits and vegetables to universally help prolong life. One must identify what is best for each individual. Studies have thus found that the Mediterranean diet for Greek women does actually act to prolong life, while for German women, who change their traditional eating habits to include olive oil and other Mediterranean food, it has either none or no positive effect. In fact, on the contrary, they were even found to have a slightly lower life expectancy. It is important to remember that diets together with genetics and lifestyle need to be balanced for maintaining optimal health.

This phenomenon is explained by the fact that as yet unknown genetic variants are responsible for ensuring that some people can use olive oil in their metabolism better than others. The variants produced by good olive oil producers is naturally found in areas where olives have been cultivated for many years, and as such their advantage has been sustained over a longer period through natural selection.

The main objective of today's nutrition research is to create customized diets and nutritional compositions for specific population groups that have the same health status and lifestyle, and who inhabit the same environment. In the future, life sciences will be able to use genetic testing to divide people with specific genetic traits into those groups. In this way we can come closer to a personalized diet.[33]

Epigenetics is one of the youngest areas of the life sciences and examines how our characteristics and features are formed from two different factors: nature, the genetic information we inherit from our parents, and nurture, which incorporates the influences of the environment on our genes, a major part of which includes the food that we eat.

Scientists have found that some of the changes in gene regulation can be passed to the next generation, without changing the information contained in the genes. These changes are called epigenetic markers. Until now it had been thought that these changes are deleted from the DNA, before they are passed on to the next generation. Now it looks like they can remain.

A joint American-European study found that prenatal experience of starvation can lead to epigenetic changes that influence a person's health in later life and even that of the person's children. The study shows that children who were born in the so-called "Dutch Hunger Winter" of 1944–45, were affected by life-long ill health and even six decades later were particularly vulnerable to heart or lung diseases, other ailments and to glucose intolerance. In addition, women from mothers who had suffered starvation later gave birth themselves to low birth weight children even though they had eaten enough. Such children were also found to be particularly vulnerable to disease.[34]

Epigenetics shows that the lives of our grandparents, what they ate, how much they moved or what environmental factors they had been exposed to, can be transmitted to us and affect how our body looks and how it works inside.

However, these epigenetic changes are variable and reversible. Epigenetic research is now trying to better understand how our environment leaves epigenetic markers in the DNA and how these positively or negatively impact on our health. Knowing the potential epigenetic effects of dietary behavior will enable future generations to have a healthy start in life and to stay healthy for longer. As a result, more research is now focusing on a mother's diet before and during pregnancy and the optimal nutrition of the child from the outset.[35]

Especially in recent decades, nutrition research has made great progress in understanding the relationship between food and health. But there are still high levels of investment needed to achieve the goals that have been set. This is especially true for the challenges facing emerging countries in Asia and Africa, as they have two simultaneous burdens to carry, namely malnutrition and overeating.

Classifications: The most important terms in brief

-omic

The ending -omics is given to parts of the life sciences which deal with the analysis of sets of similar individual elements, for example when looking at the genomics of the human genome, which is the totality of all genes. Metabolomics studied the metabolome, which is the totality of all metabolites (the intermediates and products of the body`s metabolism) of a human being. The microbiologist is interested in the microbiome, which is all the microorganisms that colonize humans, whether they be intestinal bacteria, microorganisms on the skin or other parts of the body.

Genetics

Genetics or heredity tries to understand the present predisposition of living human beings through their genetic makeup. It deals with the laws and material bases of the formation of hereditary characteristics and the transfer of genetic material to the next generation. The founder of genetics, the Augustinian monk and teacher, Gregor Mendel, applied systematic crossing experiments with peas between 1856 and 1865, which he carried out through statistical evaluations in the garden of his monastery.

Molecular Genetics

Molecular genetics was established in the 1940s and focuses on the molecular basis of heredity. These include the structure of the molecular carrier of genetic information (DNA), duplication (replication) of these macromolecules and the changes occurring in the subsequent information content and the realization of the genetic information in the course of a gene's expression.

Epigenetics

Epigenetics examines mechanisms and consequences of heritable chromosomal modifications that are not based on changes in the DNA sequence. This focuses on understanding the genetic regulation of development and disease processes. Epigenetic codes structure the chromosomes that control gene activity and ensure in many parts of the genome that large genomic regions remain muted. However, these codes are potentially reversible and can therefore in the course of a life be changed developmentally and environmentally. Therefore epigenetics makes it possible to observe the impact of environmental changes on genes and to understand their long-term consequences for humans.

Molecular Nutrition Research

Molecular Nutrition Research studies molecular processes involved in nutrient and micronutrient uptake, transport and metabolic, immunological and physiological response at both cellular and whole organism level. Current work in this research area investigates molecular mechanisms linking intracellular nutrient/micronutrient concentrations with an impaired phenotype (a set of observable characteristics) and biological function of different cell types and organs.

Nutrigenetics

Nutrigenetics examines the relationship between nutrition and genetics. Its particular focus is on how diet related diseases and other processes in the organism are affected through genetic variation. There are approximately ten million genetic variants and nutrigenetics studies how genetic predisposition can influence and affect dietary choices. Nutrigenomics asks how nutrition modulates gene expression. The aim of research in this area is to develop food that can be used as preventative medicine and in the treatment of diseases.

CHAPTER 2:
FROM THE BEGINNINGS OF INDUSTRIAL FOOD PRODUCTION TO TODAY

The development of the food industry is a success story with a measurable positive impact on people. The progress made to date is evidence that this industry is able to handle future challenges.

The decision about which foods were produced and in what quality was until the beginning of the 19th century entirely in the hands of large landowners, farmers and local food artisans such as millers, bakers and butchers. For the rural population, self-sufficiency was in the foreground, before cattle dealers and grain traders took over supplying the cities. Many farmers in the immediate area around the cities sold their surpluses in regional markets or supplied grocers and small shopkeepers.[1]

Cities with more than 2,000 inhabitants were supplied from the surrounding area in a radius of 30 kilometers with food. Large cities with more than 5,000 inhabitants needed a river or sea port in order to supply themselves. The only means of transportation on land were horse or ox carts, which had a daily range of 40 kilometers on a few then still unpaved roads. The transport of goods, especially bulk commodities, over long distances intensified and prices were reduced with the expansion of the railway network.

Before industrialisation, the food supply of cities was highly uncertain. The quality of the food obviously left much to be desired. Fraud and forgery were also commonplace. Food regulations increased in detail with the aim of protecting citizens against health risks from tainted food or misleading information.[2]

Until the early 19th century, the proportion of people living in cities was between nine to 14 percent of the world's population depending on the region. In the newly industrialized regions city population grew explosively between 1800–1914 to 212 million people. Nearly half of people working in the cities at that time were employed in industry.[3] So it is no wonder that traditional agricultural and artisanal food production was no longer sufficient to supply such numbers. Industrialization was the basis for numerous inventions and new scientific insights. The end of the 19th century saw increasing competition between manufacturers. At the same time there were still numerous cartels. Branded goods emerged which were advertised. In principle, from 1900 onwards all the structures were in place that we associate today with the production of food.

When the specter of hunger dominated the world

"The diet of the masses deteriorated continuously to a low by about 1800: Before products such as the potato or coffee and new production processes like brandy distillation spread to Europe to become part of peoples' diet, daily survival was the main concern".[4]

Hunger was so for most people in Europe until the middle of the 19th century a recurring, everyday companion. Except for the new States in North America this was probably the case for all the peoples of the world. Now as then, wars, natural disasters and climatic anomalies such as drought or too much rain at the wrong time were the main causes of hunger. However, bad political decisions also repeatedly caused famines.

The biggest natural disaster that resulted in famine in large parts of North America and Europe was the eruption of the Tambora volcano on the Indonesian island of Sumbawa in 1815. The eruption threw well over 160 cubic kilometers of volcanic material into the atmosphere, with ash and sulfuric acid aerosols spreading across the globe, causing the average temperatures in 1816 worldwide to fall by three degrees Celsius. Chaotic weather conditions, crop failures and famines were subsequently the result. The after-effects of the volcanic eruption caused the deaths of at least 71,000, and 1816 was deemed the "Year Without a Summer".[5]

Another great famine occurred in Ireland in the years between 1845 and 1852. On the one hand the aftermath of the volcanic eruption of 1815 did not impair the growing possibilities of potatoes that were the staple diet of the Irish at that time. When the pathogen of the potato blight was introduced from North America, large parts of the population lost a staple food which they needed to survive.[6] The problem was exacerbated by politics. Overall, one million people died in Ireland as a result of famine, which was about twelve percent of the Irish population. Subsequently, two million Irish emigrated.

The famine during World War I in Germany is one of the worst of the 20th century in Western Europe.[7] Germany had not prepared for a war that would last longer than a few months. There was a shortage of food that could not be compensated for by rationing or by stretching out the supply with substitutes. Acorns, straw and even sawdust were processed to create bread. Almost the entire German population suffered from malnutrition, as staple foods were rationed from 1915.

The name given to the infamous "turnip winter of 1916/17" reflects the fact that for much of the population the turnip became the main food. It was processed in all possible ways, as a soup, as cutlets, as a pudding, as jam, and as bread. In Germany probably 800,000 people died between 1914–1918 from hunger and malnutrition. Many staple foods remained sparse even after the end of the war and the rationing of food supplies only reached the pre-war level by 1924. Today this term has largely fallen out of use in Germany.

After World War II in China there was a great famine between 1958–1961, which was both due to bad weather as well as the policies of the Communist Party. In this period they sought to catch up with western industrialized countries by initiating the "Great Leap Forward." This included a forced collectivization of agriculture which created the additional burden of farmers cooperating in industrial projects.

Three quarters of the Chinese population were still working at the time in agriculture which was mostly based on small plots tended by hand. As more farmers moved from the countryside to the cities there was a decrease in agricultural yields. At the same time the grain the farmers produced was seized for export. According to Chinese government statistics around 15 million people died in the four years of malnutrition that followed. Unofficial estimates put the number of deaths by starvation at between 20 to 45 million.[8]

Population growth and food shortages

From the mid-19th century in Europe and North America there was not just a focus on feeding larger parts of the population by increasing agricultural production. Food should also be safer and healthier. But up to that point, the transition from feudal agriculture to industrialization for many people was connected to social decline. "The poor usually could still afford meat, bread and vegetables in 1500, but the position of the lower layer of society in the early industrial period deteriorated further. The Pauper (lat. Pauper = poor) survived in 1830 on no more than a diet of potatoes, rye bread, coffee and brandy".[9]

In 1750, the world population stood at 629–961 million,[10] with around 160 million people in Europe. Since then, the number of people in Europe increased steadily. The reason was that more people survived to reach a marriageable age and the birth rate increased.

However, agricultural yield increases did not keep up with population growth. By growing potatoes significantly more food energy was produced from the same acreage as grain production, but that did not change the poverty of the rural population. Through the clash of old feudal structures in the country and new modes of production in the cities, the phenomenon of "pauperism" arose in Europe, a structural, longer-lasting and widespread poverty that was neither explained by individual behavior nor attributed to one single cause.

In the pre- and early industrial era home industries played a big role. The introduction of factory work, changed both the familiar structure of the factory workers as well as their concept of time. "By around 1850 reducing costs meant simple households could afford to be self-sufficient. But the general impoverishment of the country limited its ability to produce nutritious food for itself ".[11] As the purchasing power of wages fell, many people had to rely on charities to feed the poor. "In major cities in the early 19th century eating food out of the home was almost the norm for the underclasses. They were served in the street by businesses offering the sale of small meals ".[12] It was still far from the ideal of the housewife who cooks for the family through home baking.

With industrialization came prosperity

Large famines reappeared in Europe from mid-19th century only in connection with wars. One reason was the fact that agricultural productivity had been increased by the agrarian revolution. Also there was a revolution in transport due to the expansion of railway networks as well as by intensifying maritime and overseas trade. In the mid-19th century, it became possible to create products from surplus supplies in North America and Eastern Europe for growing industrial cities. Through new conservation methods and the onset of the industrial processing of foods these were also more durable with better storage and transportation.[13] There was more cheap food on the market. Nevertheless, there were still parts of the population that up to the end of the 19th century in Europe were poor or malnourished.

The food industry was developed in the 19th century through several different scientific and technological developments. Scientists like Louis Pasteur and Justus von Liebig provided the essential foundations and impulses of industrial food production with their research and discoveries. The pharmacist and businessman Henri Nestlé is one of these still unforgotten personalities. Another strong impulse came from the development of artisanal methods of food processing to industrial processes on a larger scale. Particularly notable are advances in meat and milk production as well as the milling and sugar industries. Among the most important processes was the preservation of food by drying, conserving, sterilization or pasteurization. But the invention of refrigeration machines to cool food or to even freeze it was one of the major steps towards the present.

The findings of scientific research and new processing facilities led to the development of numerous food products that had not yet or not previously existed in this form and quality. These included, for example, meat extracts, infant cereals, condensed milk, margarine, milk and melting chocolate and instant coffee. But it was not only important to produce new products using new methods, but this market as well created products with mass appeal, synonymous with names such as Maggi, Kellogg's, Heinz, Libby's, Campbell or indeed Nestlé.

Personalities made history

Justus von Liebig (1803–1873) was neither an industrialist nor a merchant, but was wholeheartedly a scientist. In 1825 he was appointed as full professor of chemistry and made his main focus research into organic substances. He developed not the new field of agricultural chemistry, but dealt in the 1840s with the analysis of meat. He came to believe that the significant nutritional value of meat lay in its soluble constituents.

As a meat substitute for the sick and poor, he steamed broth into a syrup from which an invigorating soup could again be made if necessary. However, around 30 kilogram of beef was required as a starting material for one kilogram of meat extract. Since meat prices were still very high at that time, this was not thought of as an industrial production initially. In the early 1850s Liebig succeeded, through the use of his meat extract, to save the life of the daughter of a friend who because of an infectious gastrointestinal disorder could not take any solid food. He published his findings in the Annals of Chemistry under the title A new meat broth for the sick.[14]

The Hamburg entrepreneur and engineer Georg Christian Giebert read Liebig's publication and offered to industrialize the meat extract process in Uruguay. In South America, there was at that time a large excess of beef because the animals were kept and slaughtered only for their hides, horns and bones, but the meat could not be used because of its rapid perishability.

In 1863 the industrial production of Liebig's meat extract started and from 1865 the company was called Liebig's Extract of Meat Company Ltd. Liebig limited his activities exclusively to checking the quality of the product that bore his name. Since the meat extract was very expensive it was at first only used as a health remedy and for soldiers. Soup bases and seasoning were soon replaced by vegetable products produced by Maggi for the broad market. However, Liebig's meat extract is part of fine cuisine even today.

The merchant and mill owner Julius Maggi in Switzerland had first made an easily digestible, high-protein and high-fat food based on legume flours, which was fast and inexpensive to prepare. The impetus for this came from the doctor and factory inspector Fridolin Schuler. He held a lecture at the annual meeting of the Swiss Public Welfare Society in 1882, on "The diet of the working population and their shortcomings", in which he recommended the consumption of legumes to ensure adequate nutrition. "A great impact on everyday fare was factory work. After all, meal times were now adapting to the running of machines. We ate early in the morning before work and late in the evening after work, which reduced the importance of the previous midday meal. The common twelve-hour working day was often interrupted by a single break".[15]

In 1883 Maggi began the industrial production of its legumes flour. Although this was nutritious, it unfortunately had little taste and sold poorly. So from 1866 he developed various dry soups and the now famous plant-based soup seasoning flavor enhancer. Its great advantage was that it added a meat-like flavor without containing animal proteins. But Julius Maggi was inventive not only in food. He also designed the unconventional shape of the product's bottle and the yellow label. In 1908 he succeeded with the invention of the stock cubes, another worldwide success. Industrially produced foods were now finally reaching the consumer.

The high child and infant mortality—in the 1860s one in five children died before the age of one year from malnutrition or diseases—also caused Henri Nestlé (1814–1890) to deal with this problem. Heinrich Nestle, or as he called himself later, Henri Nestlé was originally from Frankfurt am Main in Hesse and worked as a merchant and manufacturer in Vevey, Switzerland from 1843. He had developed a "soup for infants", which had been invented by Liebig but was very expensive to produce and sold only in pharmacies. He himself said that this was not a new discovery, but a real and rational use of substances which were known to be beneficial for the infant. Milk, bread and sugar of the highest quality were the main components.[16]

First, a biscuit-like easily digestible bread was made, which was then crushed into powder and mixed with a paste of milk and sugar. This mass was dried and potassium bicarbonate was added to promote wholesomeness. The resulting powdery "kids meal" was made into a liquid again by adding water. Originally Nestlé only thought to feed this to children that were a few months old. But in 1867 he was asked by his friend Professor Shredder to test his infant cereal on a

15 day old child who took neither milk nor other food. He was able to save the life of this child.

From 1868 Nestlé offered his infant cereal in Switzerland and after a few years it was available in Europe and worldwide. Since he was fully convinced of his product from his experience, he also sent samples directly to doctors and pharmacists, so they could form their own impression. In 1871 Henri Nestlé's operation employed 30 workers and produced 800–1000 boxes per day of infant cereals. The demand for the product constantly increased and in 1873 already 500,000 cans of infant cereals have been sold.

The company had now reached a size that Henri Nestlé could not run it alone in his advancing age. In 1875, the company was thus handed over to three local entrepreneurs for one million Swiss francs and the new company Farine Lactée Henri Nestlé was founded. Henri Nestlé had sold not only the factory but also its name and trademark. Therefore, his name and his development of the hallmark of a bird's nest still exist today.

Soldiers need long-lasting food

A very significant impetus to the development of new processes and products came from the military. To supply his soldiers with food, in 1795 Napoleon offered a prize of 12,000 gold francs for the invention of a method for preserving food. The prize was won by a Parisian pastry maker and confectioner, Nicolas Appert. In 1804 he combined creating a vacuum with a method of steam cooking by heating food in hermetically sealed champagne bottles and thereby conserving them.[17]

In 1809, the sailors of the French Navy were the first to enjoy meals conserved using these new methods. Until then preservation had only been by drying, smoking, salting and pickling, and by inserting food in vinegar, alcohol or sugar.

Cans conquer the market

In England in 1810 the French merchant Peter Durand then invented the can made of sheet metal, in which one could preserve food using the method developed by Appert. Durand sold his patent in 1812 to Bryan Donkin and John Hall, and the first sheet cannery in the world was founded.[18] In Germany, in 1845, the Braunschweiger master tinsmith Heinrich Züchner began to conserve asparagus in home-made tin cans. Overall, the canning industry did not develop in Germany as rapidly as in the US, although demand rapidly increased across the military side alone.[19]

Outside the US, the can was well established by the end of the 1920s. In America, it had already been fully integrated due to the fact that branded products were manufactured very early there and carried a very clear promise of quality while they were also heavily promoted. In Europe, canning compared to other food preservation was significantly more expensive and almost unaffordable for many segments of the population. There was also widespread distrust regarding industrially produced food in cans, because you could not see what they contained and check the quantity or quality. Moreover, improper processing led to lead poisoning or food contaminated by bacteria.

Canned foods were a product of incipient industrialization and in Europe were becoming increasingly important. This was partly due to the innovations in the preservation technique, such as the use of antiseptic preservatives. But also other technical improvements, such as the use of large drying equipment and freezing techniques. Thanks to them the demand for food increased which could be stored without significant loss of nutritional value and taste and consumed quickly when needed.[20]

The company Libby's was founded in 1868 by Archibald McNeill and the brothers Arthur and Charles Libby. Its first product was "Libby's Corned Beef" in the famous upwards tapering trapezoidal shaped can. Then around 1900, canned vegetables and pickles were also introduced into their range. From 1910 pineapple from Hawaii was offered[21], with canned fruit becoming increasingly important.

Another success story is the founding in 1869 of the Campbell Soup Company. The fruiterer Joseph A. Campbell and the refrigerator manufacturers Abraham Anderson, produced primarily vegetables, soup and canned meat. In 1897, the food chemist John T. Dorrance, who had studied at the University of Göttingen, developed for Campbell a process for the production of soup concentrates that contained only half as much water as the previous products.[22] Soups were at that time in Europe more popular in preserved form than in the US. However, that changed following the introduction of Campbell's products which in 1898 received their characteristic red and white label and were offered at a low price of ten cents per can. Certainly the advertising of Campbell contributed to the success of the product. After receiving a gold medal in 1900 at the World Exhibition in Paris, this label remains emblazoned on all its cans.

In 1876 the American businessman Henry John Heinz founded, together with his brother and a cousin, the F. & J. Heinz Company. He developed a secret recipe that to this day has remained unchanged for tomato ketchup. In production it used only ripe tomatoes and vinegar as the main components. The result was a pure and tasty product from the best natural ingredients. Heinz did not use tin cans, but hexagonal glass bottles and jars, in which he offered cucumbers and other pickled vegetables.[23]

Together with other industrialists in the US Heinz fought for a law prohibiting false labeling and inaccurate advertising claims and the addition of certain chemical additives in food. In 1906 the first purity regulations were adopted for food in the US under the "Federal Food and Drugs Act". At this time, the food industry in the United States had long since become an industrial leading sector, dominated by meat processing and the milling and sugar industry monopolies. It was certainly in the interest of the cartels to expand their market power through monitored quality and consumer protection. Small and medium enterprises often did not have enough capital to be able to invest in modern hygienic production methods.

Because one could not trust industrial preservation in many European countries and preservation through canning in the home was very expensive, alternatives were sought. It turned out that, glass production was able to provide suitable containers. In the 1880s the Gelsenkirchen chemist Rudolf Rempel developed special glasses for canning whose rounded edges were sanded smooth and sealed with rubber rings and metal lids. He also developed special clamps to keep them closed during cooking. His first customer was Johann Weck, who on Rempel's death in 1893 acquired the patent and exclusive right to sell his glasses and equipment. Together with the merchant Georg van Eyck he founded the company Öflingen J. Weck and Co. in 1900. Since then, in Germany the word for canning (einmachen) incorporates the company's name (einwecken).[24]

This development was also related to the new role of women in the lower middle classes. The ideal housewife was no longer working, but cared for the family and home and needed to economize and plan. After industrialization tenements lacked both space and safety for cooking. This only changed with the introduction in North America of cast iron economy stoves. In connection with enamelled cookware they revolutionized kitchen equipment.[25] The emerging cook and maid schools aimed to improve the nation's food supply and gave women their supposedly natural role.[26]

Major advances in the dairy products industry

With the discovery of the bacteria responsible for lactic acid fermentation in 1857, the French microbiologist Louis Pasteur was able to prove his conjecture that fermentation was a dependent on a living cell process. He also provided evidence that a majority of the germs are killed by the heating of food. Based on his observations, in 1888 he developed a method for killing microorganisms using heat, called pasteurization.

In the US, the introduction of pasteurization and stricter sanitary regulations led to the concentration of the process among producers. Between 1880 and 1923 the number of milk, cheese and butter sellers in Boston went from 1,500 to 131. In Milwaukee, the number of farms decreased in five years after the introduction of pasteurization from 200 to 32, and 85 percent of the milk in the 1930s came from only two companies, Borden and National Dairy Products.[27]

The research group Alpura AG, which was a subsidiary of Ursina AG (later Ursina Franck) in Konolfingen, between 1948 to 1952 developed a new method for producing germfree, aseptic milk. The process was hailed in the press as a "global sensation". The so-called UHT milk was given a significantly longer shelf life than the previously known pasteurized milk and came completely free of costly cold storage. In 1971 Nestlé took over Ursina Franck AG.

Heating is still next to homogenization the main centralized procedure in milk processing. It has been continually improved and adapted for different purposes. Raw milk has no nutritional advantages over heat-treated milk. Largely untreated milk that has only been filtered may be contaminated with germs but that depends on the sanitary conditions of the processing, which already begins during milking. Therefore, in the European Union special hygiene requirements were introduced, while raw milk and raw milk products are completely banned in the US.

The global importance of the dairy industry should not be underestimated. It is an essential component of the global food system, and with about one billion people who work in this area, it also has a key role in the context of sustainable development particularly in rural regions.

In 2011, milk production amounted to 748.7 million tons worldwide. Of this amount, 620.7 million tons of cow's milk was produced by 260 million cows. In 2010 the proportional share of milk in the gross production value of all agricultural products was 8.9 per cent worldwide. The value of trading in the global market for milk products, including aggregates containing milk, cream, butter, cheese, whey, butter milk, milk powder, yogurt and casein was estimated by the FAO in 2011 at 64 billion US dollars. Adding lactose and infant formula, the total value reaches 69 billion US dollars. According to the forecasts of the FAO and the Organisation for Economic Cooperation and Development (OECD), the consumption of milk and milk products by 2021 is expected to increase 20 percent or more.[28]

The idea of removing water from milk and then filling cans with condensed milk, also goes back to Nicolas Appert using his 1804 process of vacuum and steam cooking. By 1810 he had already written an outline for the production of condensed milk, which finally came to fruition in 1827. The process for the industrial production of condensed milk was patented by the American Gail Borden on August 19th, 1856, and in the same year he founded Borden Milk Products LP.[29]

As with Justus Liebig and even with Henri Nestlé, it was the search for responses to very personal experiences that led Gail Borden to look for new solutions. During a trip to Europe in 1851, some children died on board the ship because they had been drinking infected milk from the galley. Borden wanted to prevent this in the future by making preserved milk germ-free.

It was the American Civil War in the United States (1861–1865) that first saw the triumphant use of condensed milk. The soldiers were given 450-gram cans of condensed milk as an emergency ration, which often saved their lives. Upon their return to civilian life they no longer wanted to do without condensed milk and this laid the foundation for the market success of condensed milk. The brothers Charles and George Ham Page during the American Civil War encountered condensed milk in cans. In 1865 Charles Page was sent as an American vice-consul to Zurich and there came up with the idea to use its many cows for the production of condensed milk for the European market. The UK in particular experienced a great shortage of milk. Charles Page asked his brother to come to Switzerland to work together to establish a company with him there that would produce condensed milk under the Borden brand. But Borden refused to pass on his trade.

Therefore, in 1866 the two brothers founded the Anglo-Swiss Condensed Milk Company and imported the necessary equipment from the United States for industrial production. A year later, 137,000 cans were produced holding a pound (lb), or about 450 g. The milk was produced from 263 cows and 43 farmers as at that time most dairy farmers had an average of only two dairy cows each. In 1875 there were only two major dairy farmers, each with eleven dairy cows. Almost ten years later, the Anglo-Swiss Condensed Milk Company was processing the milk from 8,000 cows and filling each year between 15 to 17 million cans.[30]

In 1875 it was decided to make the cans themselves because it was cheaper, and in 1878 the Page brothers created their own ice factory in order to produce the raw materials for the cooling process. George Page insisted early on that his suppliers be familiar with improved hygiene rules to compete with the higher quality cans of his precursors.

Due to the great success of the sale of infant cereals the Anglo-Swiss Condensed Milk Company launched in 1877 the production of baby food. In return, the company Farine Lactée Henri Nestlé in 1878 started the production of condensed milk. Both companies were now in direct competition, but they were never really successful with the competing product. Early on they thought about merging the two companies, but George Page opposed this throughout his life. Only after his death in 1899 did negotiations begin, but the first ones failed. In 1905 it was finally achieved and the two companies merged, and although the Anglo-Swiss Condensed Milk Company was the larger company, the name Nestlé was put forward as the company name.

In 1911, the Nestlé & Anglo-Swiss Condensed Milk Company opened in Australia what was to be the largest factory for producing sweetened condensed milk. Of course, the soldiers of all the countries participating in the First World War were supplied with condensed milk.

The milk from Borden and Anglo-Swiss was protected from premature spoilage by sugar; hence, the specific technical term used for this type of condensed milk is "sweetened condensed milk". The product is significantly thicker than condensed milk, with no added sugar and a little darker in color. From 1894, the Anglo-Swiss company sold unsweetened condensed milk under the brand name "Viking" which had to be sterilized.

Dried mild powder was also an import product alongside condensed milk. Whole milk has a water content of about 87.5 percent and this was first reduced by evaporation to 50 percent and then reduced by different drying methods to about three percent. The development and advancement of the dehydration process and the transfer of these technologies were a mainstay in the development of Nestlé. In 1920 Nestlé acquired the rights to the technology developed in 1916 as the Egron method for the production of milk powder. The spray drying process was a key technology in the manufacture of Nescafé from 1938.

Completely new products come on the market

Military again played a major role in the development of new cost-effective and more durable food in Europe in the second half of the 19th century. The aim was to supply the soldiers on the battlefields. In France in 1869 Napoleon III demanded that the chemist Hyppolyte Mège-Mouriés look to provide soldiers with a durable substitute for butter. This spread was to be cheaper than natural butter, yet tasty and nutritious. It also had to be free of harmful ingredients. The result was margarine (known also as Olegomargarine, from the Latin oleum = oil and Greek márgaron = pearl), a mixture of beef fat and milk. Margarine acid was discovered by the Paris chemistry professor Michel Eugène Chevreul through his research on beef fat in

1819. As there were pearl-like shining crystals in the test tube, this led him to choose the Greek word for pearl for his discovery.[31]

Two years after Mège-Mouriés created a "margarine Mouriés" patent in 1869, he sold it in 1871 to the Dutch butter merchant Jurgens. They established in the same year in Oss in southern Netherlands a margarine factory. His fiercest competitor, the butter merchant Hongda, did exactly the same. In 1888, the two entrepreneurs established separate margarine factories in the Lower Rhine region in Germany. The reason was that the import of margarine had been given a 30-percent protective tariff.

In the subsequent years, Jurgens and Van den Bergh were the leading margarine manufacturers in Europe. In 1927 they merged their businesses to create Margarine Unie N.V. based in Rotterdam. At the same time in England the Lever Brothers company produced and marketed a "kunstbutter" under the brand name "Butterine", which was also distributed in the USA and Commonwealth countries. In 1930, the company Margarine Unie and Lever Brothers combined to form Unilever N.V. in the Netherlands and Unilever in London, creating the largest ever merger in the world at that time.[32]

Between 1866/1867 the Berlin chef Johann Heinrich Grüneberg developed the so-called "Erbswurst" and sold the idea to the Prussian army. With the Franco-Prussian War of 1870/71 the troops were supplied with Erbswurst which is a dried soup consisting of pea flour, fat, bacon and spices. To prepare it one first dissolved the dry extract in cold water before heating it. The name Erbswurst arose because the ingredients were initially pressed and portioned by hand in a natural casing. From 1922 the sausage casings were replaced by greaseproof paper as a packaging material. The manual packing process was only replaced in 1950 by wrapping and tying.[33]

From 1889, Erbswurst was produced by Knorr in Heilbronn. Knorr was founded by Carl Heinrich Theodor Knorr (1800–1875) as a grocery store. In 1873 the founder and his two sons experimented with legume flours to produce a dry soup in a mixture with dried and ground vegetables and spices that could be prepared quickly. After the death of the founder, the company was named "C.H. Knorr–granulators, agricultural products, soup ingredient factory". Since 2000, the Knorr brand has been part of the Unilever Group.

The importance of the food industry is growing

The combination of agriculture, industry and transport revolution, produced a structural model for the food industry in the US, which also served as a model for Europe before the First World War. In the US, wheat cultivation spread westward, as with pigs and corn. In Chicago and Kansas City, a meat industry of hitherto unknown dimensions emerged. Vegetables came from the south and fruit from California.[34] By 1900, the production of food had become a leading industrial sector in the US. It included the most important areas of meat processing, the milling industry, the sugar industry and the production of bakery products.[35]

American food manufacturers were larger than those in Europe and also had higher market shares. Most large companies were created between 1870 and the First World War and had developed especially successful products or even entire product groups. But even in Germany the food industry had since 1895 occupied second place behind heavy industry (mining and steelmaking). Since food production required large amounts of capital, it was raised the same way as did railway companies, namely in the form of joint stock companies.[36]

The discovery of beet sugar

No other staple food is so connected to the 19th century industrialization as that of sugar. For centuries sugar was extracted from sugar cane as a luxury item. This only changed when in 1747 the Berlin pharmacist and chemist Andreas Sigismund Marggraf discovered that you could extract sugar from white beet. A student of Marggraf, Franz Karl Achard began to grow sugar beet near Berlin and then in Cunern in Silesia built the first sugar beet factory in the world. There it was able to process 3,600 beets per day in a "factory" that counted only 13 employees.[37]

But cane sugar remained the preferred product. That only changed in 1806 when the continental blockade by the French of English imports obstructed the trade in cane sugar. By 1850, in Europe so many beet sugar factories became established that the price of sugar fell and sugar itself became an everyday product. Thanks to the abundance of sugar production a sugar processing industry quickly arose.

Chocolate—a tempting product

Since sufficient sugar was available cocoa could be mixed with it to produce chocolate. By the beginning of the 19th century this was mainly consumed dissolved in drinks. The manufacture of a specific cocoa beverage was only possible with the invention by van Houten (1830) of cocoa powder.

In 1819 François-Louis Cailler in Corsier-sur-Vevey first produced his own chocolate and soon moved production to a new factory. By 1826, the Swiss chocolate entrepreneur Philippe Suchard had invented a machine for the mixing of sugar and cocoa powder, called Mélangeur. As a consequence Cailler decided to move from artisanal to industrial production as well.

The sons of François-Louis Cailler established their father's business in the rue des Bosquets in Vevey. The daughter of the company founder Fanny Louise in 1863 married the candle manufacturer Daniel Peter, whose business was deteriorating due to the growing use of kerosene lamps and therefore he substituted his business with the chocolate shop. In 1867 he founded Peter-Cailler et Compagnie. After discussions with his friend Henri Nestlé, he tried to create a new product by combining milk and chocolate. In 1875 he finally succeeded to produce milk chocolate from cocoa, sugar and condensed milk, which was well received by customers.

In 1878 Daniel Peter's product was not only awarded prizes, but also exported to London.[38] After this came hot chocolate in powder form, the first combination of milk and cocoa in a product, and a little later he succeeded in making solid milk chocolate in block form. This would soon seduce the world.

In 1879 the Swiss chocolate manufacturer Rodolphe Lindt created a special stirring machine, the Conche, which gave the chocolate its well-known melting character. Meanwhile, in Switzerland next to Cailler, Peter, Suchard and Lindt chocolate there were numerous other smaller producers, including the company run by Amédée Kohler. In 1904 the firm of Kohler was merged with the Peter company to produce the Société Générale Suisse de Chocolat. In the same year this company started to produce chocolate for Nestlé and to sell it under the Nestlé name and through its distribution system.

In 1911 Peter, Kohler and Cailler formed a company together called the Condensed Milk Co. in which Nestlé and Anglo-Swiss held 39 percent in shares, before 1929 saw a final merger between Nestlé and Cailler, Peter and Kohler. The products were still sold under the brand names Peter, Cailler, Kohler and Nestlé.[39]

But the real triumph for chocolate only came after the Second World War. As price competition among manufacturers increased there was a concentration of a few big producers. A relative reduction in prices helped the spread of its consumption.

Cold Preservation

That food lasts longer if it is kept cool has been known for thousands of years. In winter ice was cut from lakes and stored in blocks in ice cellars or ice warehouses. As industrialization increased so did the demand for ice in slaughterhouses and breweries, as well as commercially.

Besides the drying of food products such as milk, coffee and soups, canning and refrigeration technology rendered the most important contribution to the nationalization and globalization of continuous food supply. In the US in 1914 the ice industry achieved an annual volume of 21 million tonnes, half of which went to households. In 1880, production stood at five million tonnes. For climatic reasons, the ice industry never reached the dimensions of the United States in Central Europe. In Europe, the cooling boom began with the specialist ice factory that then with the introduction of electric refrigerators again lost its importance.[40]

The basis of modern refrigeration technology was established in 1876, when Carl von Linde (1842–1934) developed a refrigerating machine together with the Augsburg machine factory and with the support of breweries. A compression technique developed by Linde subsequently went on to conquer the world. In industrialized regions specialist ice factories and cold stores were now being built in large numbers to supply the growing population with fresh food.[41] A short time later cargo ships were also equipped with refrigeration facilities to transport fresh meat from South America to Europe. England was one of the main importers of frozen meat for Europe. Since the United States could not satisfy the need for strong domestic demand, Argentina, New Zealand and Australia came into the picture. The important thing was now to organize a closed cold chain to transport the chilled food over long distances.

Even wealthy households as part of the growing prosperity equipped themselves with iceboxes for natural ice. The ice was contained at the top, while walls isolated it from the stored food, and the lower part had a melting tank. Such refrigerators consumed an average of eight kilograms of ice per day. The price of a hundredweight of natural ice in Germany in 1900 was around 50 pence, which corresponded to two to three hours wages for an artisan. Although the first electric refrigerators in the USA came on the market in 1910 and quickly found acceptance there, in Europe the use of artificial ice especially for the operation of refrigeration facilities in stores and in restaurants was the preferred cooling method. But private consumers also kept using them because of the cheaper cost up until the 1950s.

The first refrigerator in drum form was produced by Robert Bosch AG in Germany in 1933 after four years of development and cost 365 Reichsmark.[42] This device prepared Bosch for its entry into the field of automobile accessories having established a footing in the home appliance market. Because of its high price, this refrigerator was sold only around 5,500 times and then taken off the market. In 1936 a successor in the already classic rectangular cabinet form, as they are known today, was produced. Overall, only 30,000 refrigerators were produced in Germany by 1935, while the two-million mark was already reached in the United States in 1937.

Only after the war did the refrigerator become a symbol of wealth in Europe. By 1960 already half of all West German households owned a refrigerator. Through its dissemination, peoples' shopping and consumption habits changed fundamentally. Perishable foods experienced a big boom and the introduction of freezer technology ensured that more ready-made products were purchased.

The American Clarence Birdseye had observed Eskimos as a fisheries biologist between 1915–1922, and the thaw in Arctic temperatures naturally meant frozen fish were available to eat as fresh fish after weeks or months. So he came up with the idea of developing double-belt freezers and is considered the inventor of frozen food. 1923 saw the first demonstration of a plant for deep freezing foodstuffs. By 1929 The Goldman Sachs Trading Corporation and The Posthum Company bought the patent and trademark rights.[43] From 1930, more and more frozen food became available in the US, especially fresh fruit and vegetables. In Europe frozen products gained importance only after the Second World War. In 1941 the Swedish company A/B Marabou bought the company Findus, which initially produced preserves and frozen products from 1945 such as spinach and green peas. In 1949 frozen fish fillets followed. Findus was taken over in 1962 by Nestlé.

The introduction of frozen food saw the popularity of frozen fish become established. This was followed in the 1960s by frozen raw products, which were in the 1970s and 1980s accompanied by prepared meals, bakery products and French fries. Today, there are still a great variety of ready meals. In 1956, Bosch launched its first freezer on the market. In 1959 large equipment was also produced for the hotel, catering and food industries, but their development in Europe was mostly twenty years behind the US.[44]

An essential element in the continuous supply of high-quality food to widespread portions of the population with was the emergence of a food market supplied by many small shops. This development in the 19th century saw the transition from a subsistence economy to consumer business. It also required many changes in people's minds. In the 18th century efforts were made by the government to restrict food consumption in parts of society, in order to achieve a positive trade balance. The consumption of food in their own country was interpreted as a destruction of value, which deprived the State and the country of wealth. This view was overcome only by the onset of liberalism in the 19th century.[45]

Only through new industrial processes, newly developed food ingredients and highly efficient logistics in cooperation with the retail sector, could the variety of products known today be produced.

What has changed since the baby boomer period

Baby boomers are the members of the baby boom generation, which in the US is from the mid-1940s to the mid-1960s and in Europe from the mid-1950s to the mid-1960s. Baby boomers grew into an affluent society that had not previously been known. In the field of nutrition both fast and convenience foods were characteristic of this new lifestyle which had developed in the first 50 years of the 20th century. But the dominant trends in nutrition were only established in the years after the Second World War. The previously developed technologies for food production were further refined, new sales and distribution forms for foods developed rapidly, wages rose and the price of food declined. Everything was in abundance and available to large swathes of the population.[46]

So-called fast food, a term which popped up in the mid-1950s in the United States in connection with take-away meals, refers primarily to the short period between ordering and consuming the finished meal. Although the term originated in the 20th century, it was developed from eating habits established in the late 19th century. Generally self-sufficiency lost importance in the major cities around the turn of the century. In simple restaurants a cold and inexpensive fast food in the form of meatballs, chops and bread was offered, for example, in Berlin. In London there were fish and chips instead. The metropolitan population increasingly replaced traditional warm vegetable food with the precursor of modern fast food. The so-called sandwich spread with margarine, butter or lard and topped with sausage, cheese or tinned fish, became the basic diet of urbanites.[47]

One of the main reasons for this development was that women as well as men pursued professional activities and so the time for housework and food preparation was becoming scarce. Nevertheless, the ideal image remained of the "perfect housewife baking at home." All over the world, therefore, fast food traditions were formed on the basis of nations' own culinary traditions.

Under the motto "time is money", the speed associated with business was also true of eating habits. The transition from an industrial society to a service society not only in the US but also in Europe, left its traces shortly after the turn of the century. Short lunch breaks no longer gave staff the opportunity to have a meal at home, because the distance was too far. Thus the demand for inexpensive lunches in a fast food restaurant grew instead. In the US, the number of these tripled between 1919 and 1929. Drugstores won an ever larger share of the fast food market which developed by around 1930 into their most important source of revenue.[48]

In the United States there is a direct relationship between fast food and spatial mobility. The automobile was becoming the dining area and the term "Dine and Drive" something of an institution. In

1921, the first drive-in fast food restaurant was opened in Dallas. A uniformed girl accepted orders and served dinner to the car. In 1964, the number of drive-ins in the US reached more than 30,000[49]. It is said that every sixth meal is now consumed in the US in the car[50]. From the 1940s, the triumph of the fast-food chain McDonald's began with its hamburgers.

The idea of selling goods at self-service machines, was developed in the 1870s in the United States. There in 1886 the Cologne chocolate producer Ludwig Stollwerck took the idea and together with the housing manufacturer Theodor Bergmann and Max Sielaff, who developed a patented coin-testing system in 1887, built the first vending machine. In 1895 in Cologne he founded the German machine company Stollwerck & Co., which took over not only the production, but also the installation, assembly and maintenance of the machines.

The company encountered many legal obstacles such as, for example, competitors complaining in court that such machines violated local trade regulations and resale bans on Sundays and public holidays. The church criticized the Sunday sales of confectionery and the possible seduction of believers during Lent, while other critics were concerned about public health.

As early as 1892 Stollwerck's friend John Volkmann produced in New York the first Stollwerck machines for the United States. They not only sold chocolate, but also chewing gum. The first machine-restaurants then emerged in 1898. Self-service restaurants enjoyed great popularity by the turn of the century in the United States. In 1929 the idea of a machine dispensing cold drinks in cardboard or plastic cups for sale was realised. Vending machines, which could dispense cans or bottles, followed shortly thereafter.[51]

Ice cream—from specialty to mass product

A typical product which can be found both in the fast-food as well as in the convenience sector, is ice cream. From 1870 onwards, you could buy it on the street in major cities from mobile sellers of ice cream. The patents for the popsicle were registered in 1923 by the American lemonade manufacturer Frank Epperson.

In the US the ice cream business was booming after the end of World War II. In 1946, the per capita consumption was already as much as it is today, around 18.5 liters. The consumers in the US remain at the forefront of sales worldwide. This is not surprising as 2-liter packs are regularly bought in American supermarkets. Chinese consumers in 2014 consumed only 4 liters of ice cream per capita, but China has now overtaken the United States with a market volume of 5.9 billion litres this year against that of 5.8 billion in the US. Germany, at 545 million litres, takes fifth place worldwide.[52]

Within the European Union the market for industrially produced ice cream stands at around 2.2 billion liters, with a market value of about EUR 9 billion. The average consumption of ice cream in Europe is 6.8 liters per person per year.

In the countries of the European Union a total of around 100 companies produce icecream. Most of these companies are small or medium in size and employ a total workforce of 15,000.[53]

Coca-Cola—from medicine to a lifestyle

In the mid-1880s the pharmacist John Stith Pemberton sought a remedy in Atlanta, Georgia for headaches and fatigue. Such medicine was usually administered, as was customary in syrup form by the spoonful. Unfortunately, this syrup was pretty inedible which is why Pemberton mixed it with soda water. This mixture was first offered on May 8, 1886 in Jacob's Pharmacy in Atlanta for five cents a glass, not as a soft drink but as medicine. Revenues left much to be desired with a sale of nine to 13 glasses per day.

Pemberton's bookkeeper Frank M. Robinson settled in the same year on the red and white lettering and the name Coca-Cola in order to offer this drink in the then popular and widespread Soda Bars. Shortly after the death of Pemberton, the Pharmacy Wholesaler

Asa Griggs Candler acquired the rights to Coca-Cola in 1888 for \$ 2,300. He bottled the beverage and founded The Coca-Cola Company in 1892. Since at this time across an increasing number of US states the production and consumption of alcohol was forbidden, Coca-Cola was able to quickly establish itself as a "substitute drug". Coca-Cola was now served not only in soda-bars, but, with the introduction of the crown cap in 1899, throughout the United States in bottles. In 1919 the son of Asa Candler, Howard, sold the Coca-Cola Company for 25 million dollars to a consortium led by Ernest Woodruff and Eugene Stetson. In 1923 Ernest Woodruff's son Robert, became President of the Coca-Cola Company. He was said to be a true marketing genius, and made Coca-Cola available everywhere in the world. Since then, Coca-Cola has become more than just a drink, but an integral part of modern life.[54]

Preparing Food quickly, easily and better

While fast food is served ready to eat or taken away and can be eaten as a snack immediately, convenience food includes all those foods in which the preparation is reduced to a few, simple steps. Even the traditional sausage was in this sense a convenience food, as is true with soup bags and cans or containers of Maggi's ravioli, which have been on the market since 1958 until today. One can divide convenience food into five different areas:

First, there are the kitchen-ready products such as uncooked frozen vegetables, frozen fish fillets or baking mixes. Partly prepared foods include noodles, which have yet to be cooked, or breaded or marinated meats, as well as frozen french fries, which are to be prepared for consumption either in the oven or in the fryer. Infused or stirred convenience food, for example mashed potato powder, is stirred into hot water, and includes all instant dishes from the packet soups to Asian noodle dishes. All precooked canned or frozen foods to be heated briefly in the pot in the oven or in the microwave can be considered as ready to cook food. The last group of convenience foods are ready to eat products. These include breakfast cereals, yogurt and ice cream, but also all forms of baked goods or fish, meat and canned fruit. Whether you still want to attribute the convenience food label to chocolate bars and other ready to eat forms of snacks or just to fast food is a matter of perception.[55]

Very important to the success of convenience foods was the contribution made by the invention of the microwave oven. Since the mid-1960s these also became available to private households. The increased sales of microwave ovens in the United States led to them overtaking gas stoves for the first time in 1975. By 1976 microwaves were more widespread in American households than the dishwasher. Today their level of use in households in Japan stands at 98 percent, in the US at 85 and Germany at 75.[56]

Two products that have changed the world's breakfast habits in the convenience sector are Nescafé and Kellogg's cornflakes.

The challenge to capture the aroma of coffee

In 1930, Louis Dapples, then president of Nestlé and Anglo-Swiss Condensed Milk Company, was visited by representatives of the Brazilian government and the Brazilian Coffee Institute, to whom he proposed making a coffee concentrate which would preserve the flavor of coffee and be easily dissolved in hot water. The background to this inquiry was that Nestlé through its dry milk products had a worldwide reputation and that Brazil produced coffee in abundance, such that the country was forced to destroy part of its crops so as not to see prices fall through the floor on the world market.

By preserving it in concentrate form it would offset market fluctuations as well as attract new coffee lovers. But the problem in Brazil could not be solved quickly enough. Louis Dapples had indeed commissioned the Nestlé Research Laboratory in Switzerland to immediately solve the problem, but a research team led by Max Morgenthaler needed quite a few years until it was able to preserve the aroma of coffee.

In the spring of 1937 a soluble powder was finally produced that could be manufactured on an industrial scale. On April 1, 1938, Nescafé was first offered in Switzerland. It was a success from the beginning. As a result more Nescafé factories were shortly thereafter established in France, Great Britain and the United States.[57] Since Nescafé was available to the troops from the US Army, it quickly attained a high profile and worldwide distribution. In Germany Nescafé has been produced since 1943, but initially only for the flight crews of the Air Force. In the 1950s, Nescafé then developed into the fashionable drink of the growing baby boomer generation. In the following decades, the manufacturing process for Nescafé has been continuously improved and a large number of variations for various flavors produced. Today Nescafé is the most valuable brand in Switzerland.

Breakfast from the sanatorium

The world's popular breakfast cereals today have their origin in the Western Health Reform Institute, a sanatorium founded in 1866 by two Seventh-day Adventists James and Ellen G. White in Battle Creek, Michigan. On the basis of their religious beliefs and the principles of naturopathy they preached abstinence from meat, alcohol, tobacco and coffee, and in their sanatorium mainly ate bread.

After John Harvey Kellogg took over the management of the sanatorium in 1876 and his brother Will Keith Kellogg also started to work there, the two brothers began to look for food alternatives for the sanatorium patients. By chance, they discovered that water swollen wheat grains could be a healthy alternative to bread by pressing and drying them. Looking to provide for a patient after his treatment, the brothers founded a mail order business. Will Keith Kellogg continued to experiment and developed his cornflakes baised on maize.

The success of the breakfast cereal spread quickly and in Battle Creek, there were soon more than 40 breakfast cereal producers. The entrepreneurial stimulus was to reduce the cost of cereals through a simple manufacturing process and produce a high-priced health food. In 1906, Will Keith Kellogg then founded the Battle Creek Toasted Corn Flake Company, which became the Kellogg Company in 1922.[58]

The popularity of Kellogg's Cornflakes is owed on the one hand to the intense and skillful approach to marketing and advertising and on the other to a change in the eating habits of Americans. Until the end of the 19th century, a breakfast of bread or porridge with fried bacon was associated with a certain effort in the kitchen. By the turn of the century, products were being sought that could be cooked faster and more conveniently. Cornflakes needed only to be poured into a bowl and topped with milk or another liquid. They were packed hygienically and through advertising became well known.[59]

Cornflakes were from the beginning associated with health having been invented in a sanatorium, and advertised to reinforce this view. Over time, more and more varieties of corn flakes, whose taste was added to by the addition of sugar, attracted children and young people.

The international food industry

In a case study of Nestlé in November 2015, the Harvard Business School examined the situation of the largest multinational food manufacturers (N 9–716–422). Most of these companies were founded like Nestlé in the second half of the 19th century or early 20th century. Due to ever improving production methods the proportion of packaged and convenience foods reached extremely high levels in the period between 1950 and 1990.

In 2013 the 500 largest food manufacturers in the world had a market share of 70 percent in the preparation of industrially manufactured foods. Based on the entire food market, Nestlé was a leader at just over 1.5 percent. The market value for food was 7,000 billion dollars[60] worldwide.

Since the mid-1990s, the company was increasingly confronted with global environmental problems and the health problems of the population, which were ultimately reflected in consumer behavior. There were quite different reactions to dealing with these new challenges.

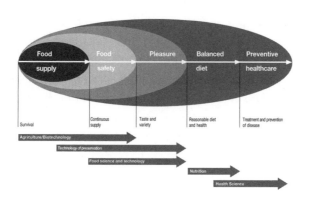

Fig. 4: The food system: from agro-processing poducts to nutrition and health

Pepsico: switch to healthier foods

The company Pepsico was by 2014 the world's second largest food and beverage manufacturer, a position achieved primarily due to numerous mergers and acquisitions since the 1970s.

In 2005, the first Sustainability Report was published, in which the company showed how it wanted to reduce water and energy consumption in the manufacture of its products. Since 2006, Pepsico's full range of products is more and more focused on healthier foods and beverages. However, this resulted, in the opinion of market observers, in a loss of market share and turnover by 2011. These decreases needed to be offset by austerity measures. Simultaneously Pepsico began to develop new raw materials for its products.

Unilever: sustainable production of agricultural products

The Unilever group established in 1929 was from the beginning not only a food producer but also a major producer of detergents and toiletries. Since 1999, the focus has increasingly been on its 400 core brands. And, since the 1990s, Unilever has consistently promoted the sustainable production of agricultural products. This saw the company secure top position in the Dow Jones Sustainability Index for food and beverages in 2000.

The goal to be the market leader in the field of sustainability was achieved by Unilever in 2010, while 48 percent of the agricultural products used by the company were sustainably sourced in 2014. The company began to lessen its focus on its food business and expand its range of personal care products, until in 2015 it was no longer classified as a food producer but as a manufacturer of personal care products.

Coke: reduction of calorie content

In 2014, Coca-Cola was the world's largest producer of non-alcoholic beverages. The first environmental report published by the company in 2002 focused on the reduction of water and energy consumption as well as on the prevention of waste. Given the global increase in obesity and diabetes Coke began in 2008 to put more emphasis on promoting physical activity among its customers. In 2014 more than 100 new products with a reduced-calorie content or calorie-free had by then been introduced onto the market. Another approach to calorie reduction was to offer smaller packages.

Mondelez: incentives for responsible consumption

Mondelez International is the third largest food producer in the world after Nestlé and Pepsico and has its roots in the company, Kraft Foods, founded in Chicago in 1903, as a cheese producer. In 1988 Kraft was taken over by the tobacco manufacturers Philip Morris, which already included the food company General Foods. Philip Morris thus became, at least temporarily, the biggest food conglomerate in the world. More mergers and acquisitions followed. In 2007 Kraft became an independent listed company and took over the British confectionery manufacturer Cadbury in 2010. In 2012 it was forced to split into two separate listed companies and led its global activities under the name of Mondelez International.

Under the motto "better choice," Mondelez also began to revise its products and to make them healthier. There were also improvements in resource use and environmental impact. With the "mindful snacking" program, consumers were encouraged to be more responsible consumers.

Danone: health through nutrition to as many people as possible

Danone is the world's largest manufacturer of dairy products and the second largest in the field of bottled water and children's nutrition. It has not taken long to reach this point. In 1973 the French glassmaker Boussois Souchon—Neuvesel (BSN) merged with Danone to enter the food market. It focused from the outset on strong brands. Initially the new company BSN-Gervais-Danone was, for a few years known as BSN before returning to the name Danone at the beginning of the 1990s.

In 1997 the company decided to focus exclusively on dairy products, bottled water and pastries. Thus Danone in the early 2000s positioned itself as a manufacturer of healthy food. In 2007, it bought the biscuit division of Kraft Foods which was enriching its products with micronutrients. From 2012 Danone then focused on four business areas, namely fresh dairy products, water, baby food and medical nutrition.

The goal of Danone was that by 2020 it would convert itself from a company producing food and beverages to a company that positively affected the eating habits of its customers. Its motto is: "health through nutrition to as many people as possible". The English key concept is: "Alimentation". Accordingly the company's commitment is strong in the areas of research and development.

Naturalness as a guiding principle

Since the 1970s, the environmental movement and increased health consciousness has led to a reorientation of marketing. For the consumer, terms relating to nature such as farmer, countryside or Bio were key. In the US in 1984 twenty percent of industrially produced foods were sold as Light or Diet products.

The function of food transformed profoundly in the face of a more affluent society. Its symbolic character increased along with it. Food was situational and an expression of lifestyle and attitude. The fact that through the industrial production of food, the health of nations and the life expectancy of the widest sections of the population have been significantly improved has been forgotten.

The development of research from its beginnings to nutrigenomics

Research and development are deeply rooted in the history of Nestlé. The "Nestlé infant cereal" developed by Henri Nestlé when the company was founded in 1867, was a research product. Research and development (R & D) in the modern sense began at Nestlé in the 1930s, when Max Morgenthaler and his team conducted research into developing the manufacturing process for the first soluble coffee, before it entered the market under the name of Nescafé in 1938.[61]

The first laboratories were established at Nestlé as part of the entire production process–ensuring compliance with the strictest quality and safety standards–from raw materials to finished products. The objects of research and development were then expanded. The focus switched to developing new products and implementing the results of laboratory experiments in industrial manufacturing processes. A key role was played by the result of the first experiments of the Nescafé development center in Orbe. The processing of raw milk and the rationalization of the production of chocolate on a large scale are examples of the impact of early research activities. Among the outstanding results of R & D in the 1950s was the development of culinary specialties, the use of new raw materials for these products, the perfecting of automation and the development of freeze-drying processes.

Coexistence of basic research and practical development

The coexistence of areas of basic research and the practical development of products and processes has thus been long established. Basic research develops scientific knowledge from which new, or improved, products and processes could be developed. The practical implementation of these insights was tested through decentralized development centers around the world, Research Companies referred to as "Recos". Each center specializes in one or more product areas and is located in the immediate vicinity of a factory of this product category.

In 1987 there were 18 Recos in ten countries around the world. In Singapore and Ecuador respectively, a Reco was established in the early 1980s, and a decade later one in the Ivory Coast. Recos in developing countries were on the one hand used to examine the raw materials such as coffee, cocoa and soy, their crops and their applications locally and to optimize their use. On the other hand, they focused on the development of local products. Part of the strategy followed by Nestlé in countries with low purchasing power in addition to conventional ones, is to make cheap products available anywhere in the world that are specially tailored to the needs of the population, so-called Popular Positioned Products (PPP).

In the 1970s this had already started with the study of diet-related diseases in society. The Laboratoire Biologique founded in 1968 in Orbe (Switzerland) conducted basic research into the area that we now call "Nutrition". It dealt with problems such as obesity, diabetes and hypertension. Later the Institute was incorporated into the Nestlé Research Center (NRC).

The rest of the basic research was focused since the 1950s in laboratories in Entre-deux-Villes in Vevey, but as the company rapidly grew it proved to be too small. So a new modern center for basic research was built in Vers-chez-les-Blanc in Lausanne. The Nestlé Research Center (NRC) began operating in 1987 and has since become the largest private food research facility in the world. Initially 400 employees from all disciplines were employed, including chemists, physicists, biologists, bacteriologists, physiologists, immunologists, Experimental physicians, toxicologists, psycho biologists, computer scientists, mathematicians and other specialists.

The scientists' aims were to investigate the effects of diet on the condition and functions of the human organism and to determine the human need for nutrients. The focus of such research was on the individual constituents of foods such as carbohydrates, proteins, fats, and diet per se, particularly in developing countries. Here the improved use of local raw materials was a major theme. Werner Bauer, who took over the management of the NRC in 1990, came from the field of contract research, an indication that Nestlé's basic research was to be more user-oriented and should be brought closer to the needs of the market.

Despite decentralization, the NRC and the Recos were directly and exclusively answerable to the Management Board at the headquarters in Vevey. Brian Suter in 1987 was appointed as the first

Executive Vice-President with sole responsibility for research and development. He institutionalized the hitherto quite loose cooperation among the Recos. In 1997, the responsibility for research and development with technology, production and the environment was gathered together by the Management Board, which was now in the hands of the Executive Vice-President Rupert Gasser.

He set to work to reduce the number of Recos, now called R & D centers, with each focusing on specific product categories. Together with Werner Bauer, he developed a concept which was to loan out some R & D centers to Product Technology Centers (PTCs). There the wide range of skills and expertise from all research areas, the strategic business units and the individual markets were combined. Thus he, for instance, bundled the entire research into coffee in only two centers, Orbe and Marysville (USA), and all the milk research in one center in Konolfingen (Switzerland).

By focusing in this way it not only increased the speed and quality of development activities, but it also improved the implementation of results in the markets. While the PTCs were centrally responsible for the Group as a whole in their respective field, the R & D centers focused more on their region.

They made sure that the food, despite the ongoing globalization, was adapted to local conditions and tastes, as well as the respective cultural environments. They were supported by the so-called application groups that have long existed in almost every Nestlé factory. Their task was to make products at its factory quickly change to always continue to adapt to local tastes and local raw materials.

Nutrition as the most important internal growth target

As early as 1997 Nestlé defined nutrition, i.e. targeted healthy eating, as the most important internal growth field and created a separate strategic business division that the CEO took over direct responsibility for. In 2006, Nestlé Nutrition has been transformed into an autonomous globally managed Division. Following the establishment of the new strategic direction of Nestlé, the NRC could now concentrate its research on nutrition. The relationship between diet and health has become increasingly important as has the development of products that meet specific nutritional needs and are at the same time high quality and also taste good. The seven priorities of consumers were weight control, performance improvement, protection of the immune system, improvement of digestion, growth and development in children and adolescents, healthy aging, health and beauty.

The task of the research was also to contribute to cost reductions, without compromising the quality of the products. As regards raw materials, the focus was in particular on optimum utilization and processing in developing countries. Subjects also included optimizing conservation methods by which the natural properties of the products could be preserved.

Changes in the environment and in consumption and the production process constituted a constant challenge for research. For example, Nestlé had decades of experience with extruder technology, which gave form to breakfast cereals, ice cream, energy bars, pasta and pet food. In the mid-1990s, researchers at the NRC developed from extruder technology a special procedure called "Low Temperature Freezing" for making ice cream, which kept the full taste and had one-third fewer calories.

In the 2000s the NRC reinforced cooperation with external institutions and companies. For example, in late 2006 it began a research collaboration with the EPFL (Ecole Polytechnique Fédérale de Lausanne) on "brain food". When searching for products with added health benefits, research moved increasingly into areas of biotechnology, in which cooperation with specialized companies was inevitable.

With the increased attention to molecular orientation the individual became the central focus. Scientists tried to understand how metabolism really worked and what role genetics and epigenetics had on it. The role of nutrients was studied further, to see, for example, why for some people a high fat diet is better, while for others more proteins are necessary and again why others need lots of carbohydrates. In addition, due to the progress of data science more information could be collected, saved and–above all–evaluated. From original scientific "expeditions" there followed many hypotheses, new analyses and new ideas.

In 2011 Nestlé founded the Institute of Health Sciences (NIHS) which has the task of providing a scientific basis for personalized health nutrition. Here the institute develops biomedical and molecular nutrition research science to maintain and improve health. The institute develops and employs quantitative human profiling, integrated systems biology and big data analytics tools. The long term aim of the NIHS is to address unmet nutritional and medical needs by developing an improved understanding of the relationships between genes, metabolism and the environment to pioneer personalized nutritional solutions throughout life.

In line with the development objectives of the Nestlé Institute of Health Sciences, the Institute's research focuses on nutrition solutions for the prevention of diseases of the digestive system, metabolism, brain health, and the situation in old age. The research results are objective and produce highly sensitive diagnostics, coupled with coordinated, scientifically proven and personalized nutritional solutions. The institute's director, Emmanuel E. Baetge, has gathered a team of senior research scientists to pursue a multi-stage systems biology approach:

- the creation and use of genomics, proteomics and metabolomic platforms for a digital molecular "health check" of consumers and patients;
- development of clinically relevant, natural cell models to simulate the molecular characteristics of the aging process and common chronic diseases;
- molecular nutritional understanding which can be exploited to maintain or improve cellular function for disease prevention;
- development of diagnostic approaches that can contribute to the personalization of nutrition strategies.

The specialized biomedical research laboratories and the headquarters of the Nestlé Institute of Health Sciences are in the Innovation Park campus of the prestigious EPFL (Ecole Polytechnique Fédérale de Lausanne) in Lausanne. This simplifies academic and scientific cooperation and partnerships.

In 2016 the NIHS and Nestlé announced a collaboration with Samsung Corp. to develop personalized digital solutions for monitoring diet and lifestyle. This collaboration will bring together nutritional profiling and lifestyle monitoring technologies which may ultimately help balance nutritional, environmental and lifestyle inputs to maintain health.

The world's largest private network of Food Research

Without integration into the global research and development network Nestlé's Institute of Health Sciences could not achieve its ambitious goals. Nestle has the world's largest private network of food research. Today three centers are the pillars of this network, in addition to the Nestlé Institute of Health Sciences (NIHS) the Nestlé Research Center (NRC) in Lausanne with branches in the USA, China and Japan, as well as the Clinical Development Unit (CDU), which has also their headquarters in Lausanne. Moreover, there are

31 product technology centers and centers for research and development[62] worldwide.

The Nestlé Research Center (NRC) still operates mainly basic research tasks. It has the job of developing scientific knowledge and new technologies, from basic Nutritions- and health research to applied research for product development and application. Researchers at the NRC are working on four main projects: "First 1000 Days and Healthy Kids, Healthy Pleasure, Healthy Ageing and Sustainable Nutrition". The Nestlé Clinical Development Unit is responsible for more than 100 clinical trials by the Group. It provides medical expertise for various therapy areas and also specialized know-how for data management and biostatistics.

Worldwide Nestlé employs over 5,300 employees in research and development. In 2014 Nestlé invested 1.629 billion CHF in research and development and registered 300 patents. In 1979, the R & D expenditure was still at 153 million CHF, while in 1989 it was half a billion francs and by 2005 it had reached 1.5 billion

It is very difficult to make specific statements about the research and development activities of other companies. In their basic concepts they are similar to those of Nestlé. However, they differ mostly due to the extent of their financial resources and by the many existing links to specific product lines. Researchers can rarely work as freely within existing corporate structures as they can at Nestlé Institute of Health Sciences.

CHAPTER 3:
HOW CAN A GROWING WORLD POPULATION STAY HEALTHY AND LIVE LONGER?

In the previous chapter we have seen how industrial production methods have revolutionized food production. Industrialization also had a profound influence on the lifestyle of people and changed their diets. New, more nutritious, safer and cheaper food from industrial production not only improved the quality of life and health of parts of society, but it also increased their life expectancy. By 1930, the foundations had been laid for a better functioning food industry and for the improved supply of food to people in developed countries.[1]

Then from the 1950s these were built upon, while new developments also brought new challenges. In 1950, we had a global population of slightly more than 2.5 billion people. In 1990 it then stood at 5.3 billion. Today there are 7.3 billion and by 2050 the United Nations (UN) expects a global population of 9.7 billion people.[2]

Given the increasing competition for land, water and energy and the scope of the expected population growth, the world needs to provide enough nutritious food to feed 2.4 billion more people in 35 years than currently. Supplying 800 million people who already do not have enough food, must be secured.

In solving these problems, the adaptation of the global food system to the economy plays a decisive role. Companies like Nestlé create added value for consumers and for society. Food production, as until now, had to not only keep up with the growing number of people, but also to make up deficits. Today, people not only expect in all parts of the world, that a sufficient amount of food will be provided to satisfy hunger. Increasingly food choices are based, once a certain income level is reached, and increasingly in highly developed countries, on quantity and choice as well as food quality.

Nestlé improves quality of life by helping provide tastier and healthier food and beverage options to help people provide for themselves and their family. The food and beverage portfolio is still at the center of the business and the strategy of Nestlé. It is the broadest in the industry, ranging from popularly positioned products for consumers with low incomes up to premium products and services.

In 1950 only a third of the world population lived in cities, but since 2010 that has risen to more than half, and in 2050, according to UN estimates, two thirds of all people will live in urban areas. Such dimensions are difficult for us to imagine today.[3] But it is not just the growth of cities that has very direct consequences for the production and delivery of food. It is also the rapid economic growth in the rapidly evolving countries in Asia, South America and Africa, which increases the income of the people living there. We will not only have to produce more and more food, but more and more that matches the specific needs of consumers.

In Western industrialized countries, higher incomes, falling prices and increasingly changing lifestyles have led to a profound change in the retail trade and out-of-home catering. The rising consumption of food has come at the same time as decreasing physical activity and has been clearly identified as the cause of ever-spreading obesity, cardiovascular disease and diabetes with all the illnesses associated with these.

The causes of excessive consumption of food certainly do not just rest with the consumer and his or her way of life, but also in the structure of the food supply. The ever-increasing competition between food manufacturers and within the retail trade as well as the providers of out-of-home catering has led to ever increasing marketing activities.

The worldwide increase in food production has not only caused health problems, but it also raises the question of the use of existing resources and the consequences for the environment, for example by increasing packaging waste. All these problems can only be solved together. National governments, multinational organizations and all of the food production parties are therefore required to cooperate.

Societal changes affect the global food industry

Already at the beginning of the 20th century physicians and statisticians in the developed countries had established a clear link between the diet of people living there, their increasing health and their longer life expectancy. It came to the simple conclusion that a person who had enough to eat and the necessary nutrients can lead a healthy life. This has led to the logical conclusion in business and politics that increased food production will lead to better nutrition and a better quality of life.

Therefore, economic and health policies focused over several decades to strengthen agriculture as the source of all food. Subsidies for improved production methods, the further industrialization of agriculture, the improvement of fertilization and pest management and optimization of plants and animals were the logical consequences, resulting from the objective of increasing productivity.

Two British scientists, Timothy Lang and Michael Heasman, from City University London termed the thought patterns that since 1950 have driven the increasingly strong development in the food sector as the producer paradigm.[4] As early as 2004, Lang and Heasman forecasted that the conditions for nutrition policy, food production and the marketing of food products would in the future change profoundly. They described three different paradigms that still currently compete against each other. These involve the producer paradigm, the comprehensive ecological paradigm and the integrated life science paradigm.

The basis of the producer paradigm is the increased efficiency of capital and labor by an increased yield from the resources used. This was made possible in particular by the use of large industrial technologies. An ever-intensified production on a large scale provides the basis for the supply of mass markets. This development is associated by Lang and Heasman often with a renunciation of diversity in product range in favor of quantity.

Overall, the connections between the chemical and pharmaceutical industries and agricultural production are becoming increasingly important. The markets that are part of the food system grew disproportionately in the years after 1950, as well as the range of goods for consumers. The trend was towards inexpensive products with a growing proportion of convenience foods. The importance of brands as a guide to the consumer rose. This is evident for example in the development of Nestlé, which through acquisitions could generate constantly rising sales figures: In 1960 Nestlé had a turnover of CHF 4.1 billion. In 1970 this had risen to CHF 10.2 billion and in 1980 stood at 24.5 billion. In 2015 sales amounted to 88.8 billion CHF.

The further development of the producer paradigm through inexpensive and seemingly boundless energy available from coal and oil supported the operation of machinery and the transporting of goods around the globe. Also, regarding the use of natural resources such as land and water, there were no limits, and this included the careless handling of waste and emissions of greenhouse gases. People's health and quality of life were viewed only as a direct consequence of growth in the production of goods and services.

Environmental aspects come to the fore

In the 1970s, a new paradigm was created, the comprehensive ecological paradigm, which also included the food sector. Society, the environment, the production of goods and people's health were considered within this paradigm from a holistic perspective. Proponents of this paradigm assumed that the quality of life for each person would rise when the whole of the framework was amended so that industrial production moved concerns regarding the ecological system and biodiversity to the center.

Based on a completely new understanding of the environment, the ecological paradigm called on food representatives to not only turn away from conventional agriculture towards "biological" farming and "biological" animal husbandry, but also to begin a far-reaching restructuring of the supply chain geared towards "naturalness" and regionality. This led in turn to a move away from global trade in agricultural commodities and large-scale industrial food production.

Other major topics concerning the environmental movement were the destruction of nature by man, the waste of resources, industrial pollution, the reduction of waste generation and of course, the reduction of conventional forms of energy production. Many of these ideas, such as energy efficiency, resource conservation and the reduction of packaging waste have long since become part of our modern economic system. Thus, for example, Nestlé in the period between 2005 to 2015, reduced energy consumption per ton of products by 29 percent and direct greenhouse gas emissions per ton of products by 42.7 percent. The amount of waste water was reduced in this period by 56 percent per ton. In 2015 105 Nestlé factories produced no waste for disposal.[5]

These developments were possible without the need for any fundamental change in the system. This also applies to the use of natural raw materials and the integration of organic food in supermarkets. The emerge of an alternative movement has grown to find itself at the center of society. That does not mean, however, that there are no representatives of extreme positions which can not be integrated.

Life Science and Health

The early 21st century saw the emergence of the third integrated life science paradigm. Like the ecological paradigm, it has its roots in the biological sciences, but unlike the ecological paradigm, it was understood, from the beginning, not in opposition to the producers' paradigm but as a knowledge-based update. It tried from the beginning to incorporate scientific findings into the food supply chain. The hitherto separate areas of agriculture, production of food and health care were becoming stronger as a coherent system. Under the Health-Science paradigm individual health became the focus of political, scientific and industrial action. Hence many new challenges arose.

In 2010, one year before the opening of the Nestlé Institute for Health Sciences (NIHS), the Fraunhofer Institute for Process Engineering and Packaging (IVV) and the Weihenstephan Science Center (WZW) under the Chair of Nutrition Physiology at the Technical University of Munich undertook a study on behalf of the German Federal Ministry of Education and Research (BMBF) of the innovation sector in food and nutrition.[6] In this study, the researchers came to the conclusion that this sector has enormous potential for innovation that as yet has not been developed. However, for this to be realised a much stronger scientific orientation of the food industry is required than has been the case before. New and future scientific findings would then be implemented quickly by industry in order to respond flexibly to market changes.

Scientists predicted that food and drink companies will be faced with a number of global and social developments in the future. The new challenges concern both the needs of society, consumers and the scientific community as well as the needs of the economy itself. Companies will, in the future, see a number of providers in competition with each other, but they will also be required to provide for the consumer and society.

An essential part of the life-science paradigm is according to the Fraunhofer study to be found on the social side, particularly regarding the demographic shift towards an older population. The specific needs of seniors require the development of new nutrition and health care concepts. In addition, due to the increasing number of single households and the changing consumption habits of mobile society there is an increased need for take-away food and convenience items.

According to the Fraunhofer Institute, the biggest challenge for the entire food sector, remains to ensure a cost effective food supply for a growing world population. Cost-effective primary care is not yet available everywhere. The growing competition between plants for food and plants for energy in the production of food commodities contributes not insignificantly to shortages and to the higher prices of agricultural products.

The overall objectives such as the conservation of resources, profit optimization, the simultaneous cultivation of food crops and energy, as well as a more efficient and sustainable food production results, on the part of the food industry, in the increasing importance of research and development in order to remain competitive. These aspects are for Lang and Heasman both aspects of the production-oriented as well as the ecological paradigms.

More research in the food industry

While large research-intensive companies in the food industry have invested (in Germany) about two percent of their turnover into research and development, in 2010 across all companies in the sector this figure was only 0.5 percent. Compared to other industries this is extremely low, and this is especially true for small and medium businesses. The automotive industry, which tops the list, invests 46.2 percent of its sales into research and development activities. Also in electrical engineering and data processing, the investment volume was 20.2 percent, well above the level of the food industry, as is the case in the chemical industry with 16.1 percent and in mechanical engineering with 10.4 percent. This is in sharp disproportion to the importance of the food sector for the labor market and for the whole economy.[7]

Around 85 percent of small and medium enterprises in the food sector are merely "technology acquisition" companies. In many cases, small and medium enterprises cannot afford to be associated with high risk or radical innovations. Moreover, new and improved food for the majority of consumers is also difficult to enforce, since it is dominated by traditions, established eating habits and strong brand and product loyalties.[8]

Among the 17 leading industrialized countries, the USA, Switzerland and Sweden stand out as highly innovative countries in the food sector and hold the top positions. Germany is only in ninth place. Here, although a total of 3,427 new products between 1995 to 2001 were introduced to grocery stores, most of them had only a minor degree of novelty. In 2009, generic products totaled 8.5 percent of sales, significantly above the level of market innovations that earned only 1.5 percent of sales. In automotive and engineering new products accounted for 56 percent of sales and in the electrical industry 41.5 percent.[9]

In the field of food and the beverage industry, the world's leading 61 companies have invested a total of 8.7 billion EUR in research and development in 2012, including 15 American companies investing EUR 2.9 billion and 17 companies investing EU 2.3 billion EUR.

Within the European food and beverage industry the sector for milk products is the most innovative, followed by finished products and soft drinks.[10]

Worldwide, the total private spending on research and development (R & D) in the fields of food and agriculture from 1994 increased from 11.28 to 19.74 billion US dollars by 2004. Research spending by food producers grew the most, from 6.02 to 11.48 billion US dollars. The total R & D expenditures in food and agriculture in 2006 amounted to 18.56 billion US dollars with the US accounting for 6.03 billion US dollars, 7.50 billion in Europe and the Middle East and Asia-Pacific region 4.62 billion US dollars. Of the 10.9 billion US dollars R & D investment in the food industry 3.27 billion US dollars were made in the United States, 3.69 billion in Europe and 3.74 billion US dollars in Asia-Pacific and the Middle East.[11] It is likely that a future-oriented and science-based food industry needs to invest more in research and development.

Food to stay healthy and fit

Today, many foods, by way of their composition and when in an appropriate diet, constribute significantly more to the health and performance of each individual, than was the case back in the early 1990s. Until then, there were only two healthy life diet rules: either "eat more of it" or "eat less of it." These rules were reflected in a variety of diet fashions that usually only brought short-term success and often were even harmful. The nutritional value of food is usually only judged by the general public on the basis of the amount, the taste and its outer appearance.

Meanwhile, undesirable amounts of food components such as salt, sugar and fat have been significantly reduced in the food that is industrially produced, while foods are enriched with micronutrients whenever necessary and useful. This did not just include special food for infants or the sick, but food frequently eaten by many people. But there is still a need for further action.

Macro- and micronutrients are essential

Food has the following functions in the human body: it supplies energy, it is one of the building blocks of the body cells, and with their messengers it engages in epigenetic functions and other biochemical processes.

The nutrients that the human body needs for normal development and the maintenance of health, are divided into the two groups: macronutrients and micronutrients. The macronutrients are proteins, lipids (fats) and carbohydrates. They are not only the essential nutritional components, but also the base material of which the human body is composed. Proteins and fats together account for about 80 percent of the dry weight of a human body. A balanced 2,000-calorie diet consists of 50 percent carbohydrates, 30 percent protein and 20 percent fat.[12]

Although water is also one of the macronutrients, it is often considered separately, since the body can draw no direct "nutritional value" from water. Nevertheless, it is both qualitatively and quantitatively the most important part of our body. Water, depending on age and sex, not only makes up about 60 percent of our live weight, we can also do without it the least. Just losing eight percent of our body fluid causes serious diseases, whereas we can spare 15 percent of protein and even up to 90 percent of fat.

Micronutrients are essential co-factors for maintaining metabolic functions. The micronutrients themselves provide no energy. They include mainly vitamins, minerals, such as calcium or magnesium, and trace elements such as iron, zinc, selenium and manganese. Although very small quantities of micronutrients are needed, they nevertheless belong to essential components of the diet, because without them many normal functions such as growth or energy production can not take place. Many health problems result from the fact that on the one hand we take too many macronutrients and on the other hand too few micronutrients.

Worldwide, more than two billion people, especially in less developed countries, suffer from a lack of micronutrients.[13] In particular, they lack iron, vitamin A, zinc and iodine. However, if the food industry is in cooperation with the governments and authorities of the countries that are most affected then they will be able to address this global health problem. Nestlé is aware of the need to contribute to the fight against malnutrition and to this end it also accepts a lower profitability.

Existing industrially produced foods are enriched with micronutrients so that they are neither under- nor overdosed in terms of food portions. Particular attention is given to children and to women of childbearing age. Enriched products like Maggi soups and bouillon cubes help in emerging markets to combat the effects of micronutrient deficiency. In Central America the Maggi noodle soup is in many places more palatable as a basis for the preparation of balanced meals. Maggi has revised its entire range so that now each serving contains 15 percent of the recommended daily intake of iron and is low in fat and free of preservatives.

It is important that the food products are widely used in the respective countries and consumed regularly. Nestlé enriches with micronutrients in particular the so-called Popularly Positioned Products for consumers with low incomes. In 2012, Nestlé sold over 150 billion servings of fortified products. In 2015, the number was already at 192 billion servings and in 2016 the 200 billion per year mark will be achieved. Another objective is the development and introduction of bio fortified crops and products, for example, with a mixture of provitamin enriched and normal maize.[14]

Nestlé has a wide range of dairy products used, in particular, to help developing countries to reduce local micronutrient deficiencies. Milk is rich in calcium by nature and can be enriched with nutrients as well. Children's dairy products provide energy, proteins and micronutrients that children need to grow. To make this accessible for consumers with low incomes, Nestlé provides them in affordable formats. Depending on the prevailing micronutrient deficiency in the region products are enriched with iron, zinc, vitamin A and other micronutrients.

In 2013 30 percent of women and children in Venezuela suffered from iron deficiency.[15] Bouillons have been found to be a good support for the micronutrient iron, offered in the form of five new enriched products. In the Philippines more than one third of preschoolers were diagnosed with anemia, which was counteracted with a milk product enriched with iron. We now know that the positive effect of iron in anemia is amplified when combined with other micronutrients in dairy products and cereal.

These fortified products, at least in a broad sense, are so-called "functional foods". Although worldwide there is no uniform definition for functional foods, the working group on the science of functional foods in Europe (Functional Food Science in Europe FU-FOSE) in 1999 published the following definition:[16]

A food can be considered functional "when it exercises a demonstrable positive effect beyond adequate nutritional effects on one or more target functions in the body, so that an improved health status or increased wellbeing and / or a reduction in the risk of disease is achieved. Functional foods are exclusively offered in the form of food and not as dietary supplements like drugs in dosage forms. They should be part of the normal diet and take effect at normal levels of consumption.

A functional food may be a natural food or a food which has been enriched, a component added, depleted or removed. It can also be a food in which the natural structure of one or more components is modified or its bioavailability has been changed. A functional food can be functional for all or for defined parts of populations, such as by age or genetic constitution."

Functional ingredients in the stricter sense currently have the largest market significance especially the prebiotic fiber and probiotic micro-organisms.

Bioactive substances in foods

It has long been known that in addition to water, carbohydrates, proteins, fats, vitamins and minerals, other ingredients are included in food. These were previously partially designated as non-nutritive ingredients and/but are now referred to as bioactive substances, if they have the appropriate properties. Although these bioactive compounds have no nutritional character in the narrow sense, they can exert a health-promoting effect. While previously we have mainly been aware of the harmful properties of non-nutritive ingredients, the beneficial potential of certain compounds has now been shown in numerous studies.

Bioactive substances include, in particular, plant materials, but also fiber and ingredients in fermented foods.[17] The health benefits of dietary fiber are based on its physical properties.

So far there is no uniform definition of "secondary plant materials". In the English science literature, they are called "Phytochemicals". The phytochemicals are substances which, in contrast to the primary plant compounds (carbohydrates, proteins and fats) play a role as, among others, defense compounds and growth regulators in the secondary metabolism of plants, and occur only in low concentrations and usually exercise pharmacological effects. It is believed that about 60,000 to 100,000 phytochemicals exist in nature. However, only about five percent of the plants on the earth have so far been chemically analyzed for this aspect.[18]

The bioactive substances include the following phytonutrients: carotenoids, glucosinolates, monoterpenes, polyphenols, saponins, sulfides, phytic acid, phytosterols, terpenes and phytoestrogens. Many of these bioactive substances are fiber and substances in fermented foods. Many of these bioactive compounds have anti-carcinogenic properties, and most also act as antimicrobials, antioxidants and are cholesterol level-lowering.[19] Besides the above, there are other phytochemicals, which can be any of the above groups, but which also exert positive effects on health.

Fermentation is an ancient preservation method in foods modified by the activity of various microorganisms. Fermentation is suitable for milk, vegetables, grains, legumes, meat and fish. Today we know that dairy products with probiotic lactic acid bacteria (probiotics) have positive effects on health. Lactic acid bacteria exert an antimicrobial effect against unwanted pathogens. They make it difficult for these bacteria to adhere to the intestinal mucosa, thus stopping them from settling in the intestine. Different lactic acid bacteria are also capable of forming bacteriocins and other anti-microbially active substances. In addition, they stimulate immunity.[20]

Clearly defined nutritional criteria

In 2005, Nestlé introduced the Nestlé Nutritional Profiling System for Nutritional product verification. This system includes a catalog with clearly defined nutritional criteria based on nutritional recommendations of experts and institutions such as the World Health Organization (WHO). These are located in the annex. Since these recommendations are always based on the total supply of nutrients as part of a balanced and healthy diet, it was necessary to define specific limits for different nutrients in different product categories, taking into account the consumption habits of different age groups of consumers.

Such upper limits have been set for energy intake, for sodium (a component of salt), for added sugars, for fructose as well as trans-fatty acids and saturated fatty acids. Depending on the product category the lower limits of desirable nutrients were added, for example, the minimum content of calcium in dairy products. A product that meets all the nutritional criteria of the Nestlé Nutritional Profiling System (NNPS), receives the seal of approval of the Nestlé Nutritional Foundation (NF). Meanwhile (2015) 81.6 percent of Nestlé products worldwide now meet or exceed the strict nutritional guidelines of NNPS. If a product does not pass a taste test to the extent desired or it does not receive the "NF" seal of approval, they are subjected to very specific guidelines for product reformulation.

To enable billions of consumers around the world to enjoy a "Good Food, Good Life", Nestlé has entered a public commitment to improve the nutritional profile of its products and is reducing the content of salt, sugar and saturated fat while dispensing entirely with trans fats. It is certainly understandable that such product revisions can not all take place simultaneously in the world. In 2014, the salt content in Nestlé products for the German market has been significantly reduced. For example, by 2013 Maggi soups contained on average over 10.1 percent less salt, and pizzas from the Wagner brand "Baking Fresh" contained an average of eight percent less.

In the spring of 2015 revised cereal products came on the market in which sugar reduction was achieved in a range between 13 to 31 percent.

For foods that are aimed at children or are mostly consumed by children, Nestlé places lower limits on the evaluation of the salt and sugar content than in products for adults. In December 2015 in 99 percent of the children's products sold, including Popular Positioned Products (PPP), the company fulfilled all the criteria of the Nestlé Nutritional Profiling System.

In the years between 2000 and 2010 Nestlé reduced the level of sugar in all products world-wide by 34 percent. This figure reflects the total quantity of sugar purchased compared to the sales volume within this ten-year period. Since 2005, the salinity in Nestlé products has significantly reduced. By the end of 2007, ten percent less salt was used in those products which consumers expect will be salty in taste. By late 2010, Nestlé was able to reduce 75 percent of the salt content of these products from what was contained in the original recipes.

Since 1999, it has been part of its product policy to limit the amount of trans fats to three per cent of the total fat content in food. As recommended by the WHO, the proportion of trans-fatty acids is only one percent of the daily energy intake. The end of 2015 has already seen 98.5 percent of related oils meet the Nestlé's policy on trans fats.[21] Since the consumer is critical of artificial flavors or colors, these were largely or even completely replaced by other ingredients from the end of 2014.

Taste must be preserved

Since the stone age, man has no natural threshold for sugar and fat. Previously, those who ate the most sugar and fat survived best in times of famine, but today there are barely such shortages in industrialized countries. Cavemen consumed 4,500 to 5,000 calories per day, while today women need 2,000 and men 2,500 calories.[22]

Salt and sugar were historically used mainly to preserve foods by removing water. They then fell out of use because of the taste. The brain needs glucose to remain functional, so we look for the taste in sweets, while the reward system in the brain also becomes less sensitive to sugar. In childhood too much sugar makes disease later in life inevitable.[23]

To reduce the consumption of sugar, food technology looks to ensure that all the sugar molecules of food reach our taste receptors. So far the level is only at 40 to 70 percent. If a level of 100 percent could be reached, this would reduce consumption of sugar accordingly. This can for example take place when the sugar is found on the surface of the food but not inside it.

This also applies to salt. Noodles should be salted at the end of the cooking process, then the salt remains on the surface. By contrast, the salt in pretzels is hardly noticed and swallowed without affecting the taste much because of its coarse texture.

In the industrial processing of foodstuffs synergetic substances can also be used that make the receptors sensitive. Another strategy is to delay or accelerate the inclusion of certain substances in the gastrointestinal tract.

In mayonnaise oil droplets may be used loaded with water droplets. While eating they are perceived by the outside world as oil droplets, when in fact water is inside. In this way we can adapt food to the changed conditions of life, without changing the functions of the body.[24] The challenge is always, in every product, to combine a pleasant taste with a nutritional composition, while mitigating the preference of consumers for sugar and salt. This is especially true in children's nutrition which is important for later life. Nestlé can say that quality of life is offered through its taste.

How the global food industry is structured

The food industry, which oversees the industrial processing of raw materials into food, is a central part of what is referred to as the holistic food economy or food sector. In recent times the concept of agribusiness or agrobusiness, has been advocated. In the US, it is described as the food system, which covers the entire supply and value chain from the farm to the consumer's plate (from farm to fork).

The European Union—outwardly strong, inwardly fragmented

In the European Union (EU) the turnover of the entire supply chain for food and drink was valued at 3.600 billion euros in 2011. Of this amount, 1.000 billion euros was in industrial production and in each case 1.100 billion euros in the wholesale and retail sectors respectively. In these, and the following figures, the agricultural upstream sectors were not included. In the EU in 2011 the food system employed a total of 24 million workers. By far the largest proportion of this was found in the agricultural sector with 11.9 million workers, while in industry there were 4.2 million people and in wholesale and retail there were 1.8 million and 6.1 million employed respectively.[25]

The food and beverage industry within the EU accounted for 15 percent of total manufacturing sales. In the EU it is in terms of turnover the largest sector in the manufacturing industry and at the same time the largest employer.

75 percent of sales of industry in the EU is achieved in the five sub-sectors of meat, "other products" (cocoa, chocolate and confectionery, tea and coffee, ready meals and sugar), beverages, dairy products and baked goods and confectionery. The remaining 25 percent of total sales are distributed among the five subsectors of animal feed, processed fruit and vegetables, oils and fats, cereals and starch products and fish.[26]

Small and medium-sized enterprises of up to 250 employees play a prominent role in the European food and beverage industry. In 2011 they generated 51.6 percent of total sales and employed 64.3 percent of all employees. Overall, the sector is highly fragmented in Europe with a few large manufacturers that operate globally, and a variety of small and medium enterprises that are only nationally or regionally active.[27]

The USA's focus on out-of-home

In 2013, US agriculture and related industries accounted for a total of 789 billion US dollars or 4.7 per cent of GNP, with farming contributing 166.9 billion US dollars or one per cent. The food and beverage industry accounted for 15 percent of the turnover of the whole manufacturing sector.[28]

In 2013 there were 16.9 million full- and part-time jobs related to agriculture, which was approximately 9.2 percent of all employees in the US. Of these, only 2.6 million were directly employed on farms. The related agriculture industries, however, accounted for 11.1 million jobs in the catering industry and other out-of-home forms of catering. Food and beverage manufacturers employed 1.8 million people, representing about 14 percent of all employees in the US manufacturing sector. 31 percent of jobs in the food and beverage industry were in the meat and poultry sector, and 16 percent in the production of bread and bakery products.[29]

The share of household spending on food ist 12.9 percent, behind residential (33.6 percent) and mobility (17.6 percent). The proportion of food expenditure has declined since 1984 by 2.1 percentage points, while the share of expenditure on housing, health and entertainment has risen slightly.[30]

The supply of global and local markets

Based on sales, the food and beverage industry of the European Union (EU) is by far the largest worldwide. At 1.016 billion euros in 2012, this was larger than the US (478 billion euros) and China (447 billion euros). In the ranking these are followed by far Japan with a turnover of 202 billion euros and Brazil with 167 billion euros.[31]

The EU food and drink industry is also the world's largest exporter with a share of 16.1 percent of total global food exports in 2012, amounting to 98.7 billion euros. Among the other top exporters were the United States with 73.7 billion euros (12.0 percent), China with 46.4 billion euros (7.6 percent) and Brazil with 45.8 billion euros (7.5 percent).[32]

China in particular took years to reach this point. In 2008, Chinese food exports were only worth 29.5 billion euros, a figure which grew by 57.3 percent by 2012. Exports by the United States rose in this period by 54.2 billion euros or 36 percent and the EU reached 86.1 billion euros, a rise of 14.6 percent.[33]

Significant differences can be seen in an international comparison of the food and beverage industry in terms of the number of businesses and their employees. While in the EU approximately 286,000 companies employed 4.2 million people, in China there were 400,000 businesses employing more than 6.7 million people and in the US around 31,000 companies with 1.5 million workers. Mexico has 170,000 companies employing 791,000 people and Brazil has 45,400 businesses and 1.6 million workers, while in India there are 36,000 companies and 1.7 million employees.[34]

Nestlé is present on all continents and in 197 countries around the world. In 2014, 43 percent of total sales of 91.6 billion Swiss francs (CHF) was achieved in the Americas, 28 percent in Europe and 29 percent in Asia, Oceania and Africa. The two major markets in India and China together comprise about 30 percent of the world's population and represent important growth markets.[35]

How the global food industry works

The starting point of food production is still agriculture based on farming and animal husbandry. If farmers are, however, to produce their products at all they need to be supplied by numerous other companies, which are also part of the value chain. These include producers of seeds, of pesticides and fertilizers, and even the producers of agricultural machines. These so-called resource manufacturers also offer feed to producers in the agricultural sector who use their raw materials, and are also the manufacturer of products for animal husbandry and animal health, and even construct the sector's livestock barns and silos as well as their technical equipment.[36]

Criticism of agriculture's upstream activities and in the production of animal food has been negative and rubbed off on the whole food system. Changes, however, are difficult to enforce, because interests at the national political level ensure that securing a supply of cheap food commodities is prioritized over environmental and health considerations.

This is where one of the more recent initiatives of the World Economic Forum has a part to play, through its "New Vision for Agriculture", bringing together as partners both global and local companies and farmers along the value chain as well as governments and civil society to deal with issues from fertilizers to final products for consumers.

The food industry itself differs according to the products being processed and the processing stages involved. In the meat industry, for example, animals are first slaughtered and cut before moving onto the next stage and finally to products such as processed sausages and ready meals that are then accessed by the consumer. Similar processing steps are also relevant for milling and dairy products using oils and fats. From the flour come pasta and bakery products, as well as other products such as ready-made pizzas. Dairies, on the other hand, deliver final products for the consumer, as well as providing downstream firms with dairy products which are then further processed into, for example, yoghurt, cocoa beverages or cheese.

In this context there are also the producers of soft drinks and alcoholic beverages which in turn collaborate with suppliers to provide, for example, sugar or juice concentrates. Fruit and vegetable production can thus go in very different ways. From field fresh vegetables to canned fruit and frozen vegetables up to the production of cereal bars, there is a wide-ranging palette. The same holds true for the fish processing. From frozen fish to ready-made fish meals to canned fish or smoked fish products, there are a wide range of different products that reach the consumer.

In addition to industrial food production there are the food craft trades, which market their products themselves or bring food retailing to consumers. The retail aspect is divided between retail chains with supermarkets of all sizes, discounters and highly specialized retail outlets. In addition to retailers, we find at the bottom of the value chain the so-called out-of-home market. This includes all types of food, but also the meals in company canteens, schools, hospitals and residential institutions. In addition there are sales through vending machines. Only after these steps does food arrive at the consumer, who then often perceives it only as a consumable, without worrying about its origin and history.

As we have already seen, the food industry is global, but also nationally it is extremely heterogeneous in terms of the various sectors and company sizes. This is also reflected in the work processes involved in industrial food production. Concerning the cost of production, the quality and need to protect the environment, the automation of each step plays an important role. In the production of dairy products, beverages, bread and bakery products, a high level of automation can be achieved due to the raw materials used. This is much more difficult in the production of meat in slaughterhouses or cutting plants and is also perceived by consumers with considerable scepticism, which carries over to other areas of industrial food production.

Demography and purchasing power

The development of populations and their purchasing power as well as social change are important elements of the business environment for food manufacturers. The expected demand for processed foods depends on income level and the lifestyle. Another key determinant in a market is the age of the consumer.

The greatest potential for population growth will be in emerging and developing countries. In the years 2000 to 2005, however, the average growth in demand for processed foods in developed countries was 2.9 percent, and in emerging markets it was nine percent. Of greater importance to food manufacturers than population growth per se is the evoluation of income distribution. It is important that both the lower and the upper income classes are offered products that satisfy their needs.[37]

Trade is gaining importance

While agriculture played a dominant role at the beginning of the 20th century in the value chain as a raw material supplier, this has shifted in subsequent decades to manufacturers and wholesalers. Since the mid-1980s, there has been an increasing dominance by retailers, in particular by international supermarket chains and discounters. Being close to the consumer, and through the selection of its product range and goods, presentation becomes decisive from the acceptance or rejection of new products by the consumer.

By European and international comparison, German food retailers are included among the most actively traded. Metro, Lidl & Schwarz, Aldi, Rewe and Edeka can thus be found among the top ten European retail companies while Metro, Lidl & Schwarz and Aldi are also amongst the most active trades globally.[38] For a long time the retail chains were exclusively limited to their national markets. But then they began to operate their businesses internationally. Among the 100 largest companies in the world in terms of turnover, there are six international sales chains that also sell food, while Nestlé is the only company in the food industry.[39]

The biggest changes in the market took place in the period between 1990 and 2005. In order to strengthen customer loyalty the dealers have increasingly launched private labels. The commercial or private labels of large supermarket and discount chains were during this time the main competitor of Nestlé and replaced the other brands as major rivals.

The proportion of commercial and private labels in the food industry in the US is less than 17 percent while in most European countries it is between 20 and 40 percent, and in Switzerland even 50 to 60 percent. Of the 100 best-selling products sold by Walmart 50 included their own-brand.[40] Although Nestlé generates only 20 percent of its sales through the ten largest retail chains, it is under pressure to reduce production costs still further through technological advances and using potential savings.

Food safety remains a challenge

The growing world population and consumer demand for greater variety in food means that supply chains are becoming more complex. In our globalized world it is increasingly difficult to ensure the safety of our food. This is not only the responsibility of governments and of national healthcare systems, but also represents a challenge and responsibility for the manufacturers.[41]

The World Health Organization (WHO) estimates that in the world today two million people die every year from diarrheal diseases mostly due to contaminated water.[42] But food contains contaminants, from harmless parasites, bacteria, viruses and prions, to chemical and radioactive substances that can cause more than 200 different diseases, from infectious diseases to cancer. Especially in many developing countries, better regulation of food safety is needed, and this requires international cooperation.[43]

The two UN agencies WHO and FAO (United Nations Food and Agricultural Organization) and the OECD play a central role in the development of policies to strengthen regulations on food safety in each country and harmonize them internationally. A special role is played by the Codex Alimentarius Commission which is jointly controlled by both organizations. The standards developed by the Commission are now seen worldwide as guidelines for food safety.

INFOSAN (International Food Safety Authorities Network), is also a joint institution of WHO and FAO, and has the task of providing information about the safety of food and helping countries implement them.[44]

The United States imports about 15 percent of its food. Therefore, in 2011 it adopted the US Food Safety Law Food Safety Modernization Act (FSMA) and since 2015 it has enforced this on manufacturers worldwide. The law aims to tighten food controls and to avoid the contamination of food. Goods that are imported must meet the same requirements as those produced in the country. If this is not the case, entry may be refused. The FSMA applies to all parties in the supply chain of agribusiness. Food manufacturers need to design their processes so that they can be traced, and identify risks. US importers are obliged to ensure that foreign suppliers comply with the standards.[45]

CHAPTER 4:
LIFE SCIENCES AND THE REVOLUTION OF BIOLOGY, NUTRITION AND HEALTH

The roots of modern health sciences were established in the 1940s, as molecular genetics became increasingly important. Accurate knowledge of the smallest building blocks of life and their relationships with health and disease paved the way to a new understanding of the complex workings of the human body. Just as Albert Einstein and Max Planck have changed our physical world view, thereby laying the foundations for modern technology, genetic research changed our image of man.

The mission statement—A personalized diet for different population groups

Every person has a unique constitution that changes in the course of his life. In principle, we are indeed all very similar, but no two people are alike. This is true even for identical twins. The differences are both genetic and epigenetic in nature and they change depending on age and on specific life situations. But similar living conditions also have similar effects on humans.

Of all the environmental factors that influence an organism, diet is one of the most significant. This realization is not new. Ever since a scientific symposium held at the Nestlé Research Center in 2004, personalized nutrition has become an integral part of the future orientation of Nestlé. The model of "Personalised health science nutrition" is an approach supported by three pillars. Nutrigenomics provides the scientific basis. The fortification of foods with micronutrients ensures the health improvement of broad social groups and in the context of health management offers individual diets.

Based on these three pillars, increasingly specific nutritional strategies will be developed in the future. But there will be no single diet that is the same for all people. Differences will be set in the future by culture, existing or preferred raw materials used, and by culinary traditions. Improved understanding of the interaction of genetic and epigenetic characteristics of people with certain foods and their ingredients will achieve some degree of personalization. Of course, there will also be very specific arrangements for groups such as infants, the sick and the elderly.

If we speak of the future as being about personalized nutrition, that does not mean that there will be a special diet for each individual, at least not in the near future. In an initial stage "personalized" could mean that people might be assigned to specific groups, appropriate diet for maintenance of health and wellbeing in order to prevent future diseases or delay or alleviate existing conditions for these groups.

So we can "personalize" but the term should not be confused with "individualized". To individualize would ultimately indeed mean that for each of the seven billion people on the planet, whose number will continue to grow in the future, a special diet plan is created. That simply could not be achieved due to quantity. But what certainly is within certain limits possible today and will still be more feasible in the near future, is, in certain populations to identify deficiencies or dispositions, which can be responded to by diet.

For example, people particularly sensitive to salt can lower their blood pressure simply by omitting salt. If this salt sensitivity is not applicable or not as pronounced, the absence of salt in relation to possible high blood pressure has no effect. Nutrigenomics increasingly therefore tries to identify biomarkers, which are indicative of certain physical characteristics during a diet change. This scientific work is the real revolution in the field of life sciences.

Understanding how the body really works

In 2001 the Human Genome Project managed to map the human genome. Scientists now had a text with approximately three billion pairs of letters, which consisted of the four letters A, C, G and T. But disillusionment quickly spread. The human genome, with only 25,000 genes, could not yet help explain why some people get certain illnesses and others do not, even if the profile is identical in identical twins. In principle, it was hoped it could help advance understanding of how a flawless genetic profile would be the basis for a healthy life and help adjust the environment to allow people to reach old age.

It quickly became clear that genes not only control, but can also be controlled. Epigenetics tries to explain how and why this happens by the increasingly important task of decoding genetic information. This offers new approaches to detecting environmental influences on the genome and understanding their long-term consequences for the individual. But Epigenetics also forms the basis for information on the development of different, specialized body cells and tissues from the original stem cell.

It hinges on the question of which environmental factors we respond to with epigenetic changes in cells without the DNA sequence itself being changed. This adaptation to the environment is what can bring the body benefits, but this is not always the case when it comes to switching errors. In order to describe the totality of all epigenetic changes in an organism, one already speaks today of an "epigenetic code", which has the same or maybe even has a greater importance than the "genetic code".[1]

Meanwhile, it was realized that what we knew until recently about the functioning of the human body was not sufficient to prevent and cure the illnesses of modern civilization. The goal is to help all people lead a healthy and a long life, and this can only be reached through the targeted application of new scientific methods and insights. And it is not only just about the human genome, but also about the role of micro-organisms.

So we know what we must now explore in order to understand how the body really works and how we can explore it. We also know that the complexity of the science and the amount of data to be processed represent an unprecedented challenge. Nevertheless, we are sure that we will in the future be able to improve our quality of life, because that vision is based on concrete scientific facts underlying the dimensions we already know today.

Genetic research looks for unknown patterns

Modern nutritional research ranges from the discovery of bioactive ingredients in foodstuffs, the study of their bioavailability and biological effects, to the assessment of the dietary needs of individuals based on genomic and genetic patterns. We face the challenge to holistically understand what food ingredients do and in what way they can affect the organisms of different people.

The approach of current nutrition research, therefore, is to identify defined consumer groups, which have the same health status and lifestyle and are in the same stage of life, to more easily define a tailor-made diet.

Previously, nutrition research was based primarily on empirical studies, whose foundations were often not sufficient. Today modern nutrition research uses the findings and methods from various disciplines of Life Sciences.[2]

Genetics provides the blueprint for our genetic makeup. This information is stored in the DNA. This genetic make-up influences our predisposition for obesity and diseases such as cancer, diabetes, heart attacks or stroke. The effect of nutrients depends on the individual's genetic makeup.

Today we know that the individual is controlled by its genes, but much less than previously thought. Some genes are not all that different from those of animals. It always comes down to which gene is turned off and on (gene expression). Here an expression of the entire process of converting the information contained in the gene is referred to in the corresponding gene. This process involves several steps and at each step, regulatory factors influence and control the process. Gene products are the results of the expression of a gene, i.e., the RNAs and proteins. The control of gene expression is referred to as gene regulation and determines whether the protein encoded by the gene is produced in the cell, at what time and in what quantity. The main function of the RNA (ribonucleic acid) is to put the cell's genetic information into proteins.

Many previous studies have assumed that the single nucleotide polymorphism (SNP) is a major predictor of genetic function, and thus determines susceptibility to diet-related diseases. In a single nucleotide polymorphism, only a single base pair within a defined DNA segment is changed. However, the predictive power of these SNPs found in the so-called "disease susceptibility genes", is relatively low when it comes to the development path of health and the onset of disease onset. So far, the SNP could only explain a small degree of phenotypic variability. While the genotype refers to the entirety of the genetic information encrypted in the genes, the phenotype is determined by environmental factors as a specific expression of genetic information.

It appears that genomic compensation around the SNPs is important, whereby the same SNP plays a role in one part of the population but does not play a role in another. Despite this knowledge, business is booming for genetic counselling. More and more companies offer the consumer risk assessment and lifestyle recommendations based on personal genetic profiling. Since these profiles are based only on the SNP set in the disease susceptibility genes and therefore only have limited significance, such risk assessment and the related recommendations have a weak basis.

The susceptibility to certain chronic inflammatory bowel diseases is associated with the SNPs, in particular in chromosomal regions, but also with CNVs (copy number variants, i.e. how many copies of the same gene are present) of certain other genes. We are not yet able to provide an extensive detailed description of the genetic background of complex diseases, though it is possible. However, it is a challenging and necessary task to prevent the pathological development of such disease.[3]

The environment determines the gene pool

Meanwhile, epigenetics has found that environmental factors significantly influence the gene pool and gene regulation. Epigenetics literally means "Over-genetics", and is the science of changes in gene expression that do not affect the DNA sequence, and thus the genetic information stored in DNA. Epigenetics includes DNA methylation patterns, chromatin structure, histone code and non-encoded small RNAs. Today we know that DNA methylation is a mechanism for the long-term metabolic programming of an organism. Therefore, early childhood nutrition plays a role in health in later life. Epigenetics may also explain why people differ despite having the same genetic constitution in their phenotype. This has been demonstrated, for example, in research into twins.

Today genetics and epigenetics form the scientific basis for understanding the different preferences, needs and reactions of people in terms of their diet. In addition, epigenetics shows how this variability can itself change over the course of life.

How genes and food influence each other

Modern nutrition research consists of Nutri (epi) genetics and nutrigenomics. Nutrigenetics deals with how our genetic makeup makes us respond to certain food components. Nutrigenomics combines genomics with nutrition research and plant biotechnology to examine the molecular influence of genes on the one hand and the effect of nutrients on the metabolism and thus on human health, on the other hand. While transcriptomics analyzes the genes that are active in a biological system, proteomics studies the proteins and their interactions. Metabolomics is concerned with the metabolism of cells and tissues.[4]

In mammals, two epigenetic phenomena have been extensively studied, the inactivation of the X chromosome and genomic imprinting. The genetic mechanism controlling gene expression depends on whether an allele from the mother or the father has been inherited. Alleles are two "copies" of one and the same gene which are found in the same chromosomes in the same place. Most human genes have two alleles, one from the mother, one from the father. When both copies of the gene are active, the system is less susceptible to malfunction. One of the two copies of the imprinted genes is switched off by the DNA methylation. Embossed genes are places of susceptibility to disease because their normal function can be altered by a single genetic event. In addition, if the embossed genes are not completely deactivated it can cause genetic events of disease or contribute to the disease.[5]

Biomarkers help diagnosis

Since the epigenetic modifications only change gene expression and not the gene sequence, epigenetic biomarkers can be obtained from the expression profiles of epigenetically controlled genes. Characteristic biological features, which are objectively measured, are referred to as biomarkers. These may be cells, gene products or certain molecules such as enzymes or hormones. Biomarkers can be indicators of susceptibility to disease and may be able to differentiate between who reacts to certain food components or not (responders and non-responders). Finally, they can discover the bioactive, beneficial components of foods. All nutrients have at least indirect effects on gene and protein expression and thus on metabolism.

Epigenetic biomarkers may have the potential to diagnose diseases in early childhood that are likely to occur in adulthood. When one is able to recognize a disease before any symptoms occur, one might be able to develop new therapeutic approaches for the prevention and treatment of disease and ultimately provide appropriate nutritional concepts. However, this requires extensive knowledge of the human epigenome, and we have still same way to go on that.[6]

Created in 2006, the international Epigen Global Research Consortium, supports scientists at research institutions in England, New Zealand and Singapore. The Consortium is a joint venture of public and private institutions and cooperates with Nestlé. The diet of mothers and infants is one of the most important research projects undertaken by the Consortium. Due to its international scope, mothers and infants are investigated in different regions of the world representing very different genetic backgrounds and lifestyles in order to find out what effect the eating habits and living conditions of pregnant women have on the genes and health of their children.[7]

The Epigen Consortium has already proven that the diet of pregnant women directly affects the DNA of their infants. For example, if pregnant women do not eat enough carbohydrates, it can result in their children being exposed to an increased risk of diabetes, obesity or cardiovascular disorders. It is therefore important that the nutritional status of young women before pregnancy is optimal. To this end, a large-scale study of 1,800 young women, who have to take special nutrients up to twice daily, has been performed.

Researchers hope to be able to demonstrate the positive impact of improved nutrition in the development of children. If successful, it could lead to dietary recommendations for the general population. It has already been scientifically proven that the diet of children in the first 1,000 days of their upbringing has a major impact on their future health.

Further studies undertaken by the Consortium Epigen provided evidence of a link between the epigenetic markers in the gene HES1, which is involved in brain development at birth, and later school performance. These findings were supported by laboratory studies. From them they concluded that brain development before birth has a much greater impact on the later learning ability of a child than previously thought. Research must now uncover how the lifestyle and emotional wellbeing of an expectant mother affects the epigenetic processes in the development of a child.[8]

EarlyBird is a research project at Plymouth University Peninsula Schools of Medicine and Dentistry supported by Nestlé. Since 2000 it has dealt with how living conditions and nutrition in childhood influence health in adulthood. The aim of the project is to identify relevant biomarkers for metabolic health. The Nestlé Institute of Health Science (NIHS) is now mainly responsible for metabolically characterizing the people in the course of childhood within this project. It will include the nutrients and their metabolites (for example, amino acids, sugars and antioxidants) that provide precisely quantified information about our individual health.

The third phase of EarlyBird accompanies the cohort of 300 children in their next phase of life. While we already have extensive knowledge about how our health in childhood, as an adult and in older age is affected, there is still a gap in knowledge about pubescence and adolescence. This gap has now been closed. But it will still be a long time until all relationships are clarified throughout the lifespan.[9]

Metabolomics—on the trail of metabolism

Metabolomics is a study related to the metabolome, which summarizes all the metabolic characteristic properties of a cell or a tissue in an organism. The metabolome is the entirety of all the metabolites, which are small molecules formed as intermediates or as breakdown products of metabolic processes. Since metabolites are the end products of gene expression and gene regulation, they can be used to describe present biochemical states, which also include dietary metabolic changes.

Numerous studies have shown that diet can lead to a metabolic imbalance that increases susceptibility to diseases. Metabolic processes run in everyone in a similar way but differ individually. The effect of all substances which are consumed depends on their conversion and degradation as well as their storage in the body. The individual versions of metabolic components are laid down in our genetic makeup, so for modern nutrition research it is important to create individual metabolic profiles.

Research by Nestlé, for example, has investigated G-proteins, which are found in all cells of the human body. Their main task is to transmit the signals from the cell surface to the cell interior. Because of the central role of G proteins in practically all intracellular signaling processes, metabolically relevant SNPs were identified in G-proteins. Some of these gene variants appear to be related to a reduction in weight. For this reason, Nestlé genotyped G-protein levels in healthy adults on a voluntary basis in weight management studies.[10]

Caloric restriction is still the only diet modification that is proven to have a measurable effect on the life of many species, including mammals. In an in vivo study, Nestlé researchers examined the effects of calorie reduction and specific nutrients on different transcript levels in different tissues. They wanted to know what long-term changes in gene expression are indicated by changes in DNA methylation. This was followed by the study of nutrient-related genes that appear to have transcriptome profiles that are similar to those of calorie restriction.

Scientists at the NIHS assume that in the future food will be able to mimic some of the same effects on metabolism as does exercise. The food components with the same cellular mechanisms that are normally activated by movement would help to maintain an even and healthy energy balance. We know that human metabolism is controlled by a "master molecule" or "master switch" that controls the energy balance of the body. This master molecule called AMPK is a key protein in each cell. It monitors energy inventory similar to a fuel gauge monitoring the fuel level in a car and tells you if you need to "refuel" your energy.[11]

The microbiome—a community for the entire life

Even before Robert Koch published his work on anthrax in 1876, it was known that there are microorganisms that are only visible under the microscope. In the past 100 years came the awareness that bacteria colonize the human body, but these are only the focus of biologists and medical scientists when they pose a risk to health. The vast majority of bacteria were considered meaningless by researchers as they were seen as harmless "blackheads" that neither hurt nor disturbed the body, but just were simply present. This view only changed when they began to understand the body not just as an individual functioning by itself, but as a holobiont or superorganism, i.e. a complex biological system with many participants, that have gone largely unnoticed since the beginning of humanity millions of years ago.

After deciphering the structure of DNA in 1953, microorganisms again became the focus of scientists, because they could be analysed in a simple way through genetic research. By the mid-1980s it was possible to access even the smallest amounts of genetic material. Now you could also explore those microbes that could not be grown in petri dishes themselves. That was far more than was ever known until then.

The totality of all the micro-organisms which colonize humans is referred to as microbiome or microbiota. In addition to the microorganisms in the intestine this also includes those on the skin and mucous membranes. The Nobel Laureate Joshua Lederberg in the early 21st century coined the term "microbiome". He took the view that a comprehensive examination of the genetic lifeform Homo sapiens is only possible if one includes the genes of the microbiome. Lederberg is quoted as saying "We need to explore and understand the microbes that we carry in and on our bodies, as part of a shared environment .... Our destiny is at the mercy of the microbes that share our bodies with us. We will benefit from a deeper understanding of how they work in and with us."[12]

Around 100 trillion microorganisms inhabit the human digestive tract alone. The microbiome of the gut is thus comprised of ten times more cells than the body of an adult human. And while humans have only about 20,000 to 25,000 genes, twice as much as a fly, the number of genes in their microbiome is estimated at around three to eight million. The weight of the microbiome is comparable to that of the brain at about two percent of body weight, i.e. between 1.5 and two kilograms.[13]

The number of different types of intestinal inhabitants is estimated at 1,000 or more. The fact that this number has not been determined exactly is because when you create classic bacterial cultures 80 percent of the species, and some suggest up to 99 percent, remain hidden. Only metagenomics puts us in a position to analyze the complex community of microorganisms. How comprehensive the relations actually are between man and his intestinal residents has only became apparent in recent years. Therefore we are now talking about a second human genome.[14]

Most people are probably unaware of how large the habitat for intestinal microbes actually is. The intestine of an adult can reach a length of around 6.5 meters. The inner surface of the intestine is 180 to 300 square meters. This is because the gut is not smooth inside, but has countless protrusions, the villi, which cover the epithelium.[15]

The bowel is encased by the enteric nervous system (ENS), which consists of more than 100 million nerve and even more glial cells. The cell types, drugs and receptors in the "abdominal brain" are similar to those of the brain in the head. Both are in contact with the central nervous system, but also different messengers. One suspects that while around 90 percent of the information from the gut are sent to the head, only about ten percent from there flow downwards.[16]

Although both "brains" are very similar, they still think in different ways. The gastrointestinal tract communicates with the head-brain via four different channels of information, the messengers of the microbiome, the gut hormones from the intestinal mucosa, the immune messenger substances (cytokines) from the intestinal immune system and the sensory neurons of the enteric nervous system. This microbiome-gut-brain axis (Gut-Brain Axis) affects not only our diet, digestion, metabolism and body weight, but also the immune system, the sensation of pain, the susceptibility to stress and emotion, mood, learning and memory. All these complex relationships are explored by the fledgling discipline of neurogastroenterology.[17]

The intestinal inhabitants and their genes could have a similarly big impact on our health as our own cells and genes. To understand what effect foods have, including the macronutrients, micronutrients and bioactive substances, and dietary fiber, it is necessary to know how and why the microbiome works in a certain way or does not. The proper functioning of the microbiome keeps us healthy. Malfunctions that are often not noticed, can lead to many different diseases that have not been previously associated with the intestine.[18]

The composition of the microbiome is different for each person. Nevertheless, people can be compared and divided by blood groups in three different enterotypes. These were named after the prevailing bacteria: There are the Bacderoides intestinal type 1, the Prevotella intestinal type 2 and the common Ruminococcus intestinal type 3.

These basic types are formed for each person by about the age of 18 and are retained in principle for a lifetime. This does not mean that the environment, diet, and taking medication have no effect on the composition of the microbiome. Rather the opposite is the case. Any change in eating habits is detected in the microbiome after two to three days because bacteria have a short life cycle. Also if one is a vegetarian or a meat eater, it can be seen in the composition of the microbiome. Relocation and travel leaves its mark in the background of the microbiome as does life in a city or in the country.[19]

In addition to disposition and biodiversity the microbiome is also decisive for the disease susceptibility of a person. But this does not depend on the quantity of the bacteria. The health status of two people may be much the same, even if carrying a specific type of bacteria in 95 percent of his stomach and only 0.01 percent of another.[20] Even if the species of bacteria may be very different, their function at the genetic level seems to be very similar. In general, people who lead a Western lifestyle have between 25 and 50 percent less diversity in their microbiome than traditional peoples like the Indians in the Amazon region or Papua New Guinea.

Different intestinal microbiomes behave like various major cities and their populations: while, for example, London and Paris represent very different cities with very different populations, they are comparable in size and the main functions and experiences are similar for both populations, for example, transport, employment, education, health and safety.

The importance of the microbiome for the body of mammals, has been demonstrated using mice experiments. At the Washington University School of Medicine in St. Louis/Missouri mice were bred which were absolutely sterile. They were born by Caesarean section and then lived in a sterile cage, which itself was in a sterile tent supplied with sterile filtered air. These mice lived as it were in a bubble and were therefore called bubble mice. Even their food was made completely germ-free by heating under pressure.[21]

Since there were no germs in their environment and in their own bodies these mice had a badly developed immune system, weaker hearts and thinner intestinal walls. Thus, although they were weaker on the whole, they needed more food but metabolised this less well. Although they ate one-third more than normal mice, they had 42 percent less body fat. That changed abruptly, however, after they were brought into contact with the intestinal bacteria of healthy mice. Within days they began to digest their food better and gain weight. After two weeks their weight could not be distinguished from other mice.

An efficient intestinal microbiome therefore helps in the recovery of nutrients from the supplied food. Since the intestinal microbes also can digest fiber, which the body is unable to digest itself, ten percent more energy is obtained from food in this manner. The composition of the microbiome therefore plays a major role in the development of obesity.

But the influence of microbes was also detected in many other diseases. Diseases of the cardiovascular system are also connected with the microbiome, but researchers do not yet know what the mechanism is. In infectious diseases, the relationships are already clear. The microbes on the intestinal wall are always in contact with the cells of the immune system and prepare them to defend against pathogens. The immune system can be particularly well trained if its diversity is as large as possible.

However, the gut microbiota also act as a barrier against pathogens, as where there are already microorganisms present, other perhaps dangerous bacteria can not settle. The problem is thus to keep the balance of the microbiome whenever antibiotic treatments are used so as to avoid killing its own benign bacteria along with the specific pathogens. This is why diarrhea is often associated with taking antibiotics. But in most cases the microbiome is very good at adapting quickly to regenerate itself.[22]

As part of nutrigenomics, comprehensive investigations are undertaken at the molecular level to understand the health effects of nutrition in the relation to the genome, the intestinal microbiome and the human host. The genome contained in the food itself is explored in order to discover the effect of macro- and micronutrients and better understand the bioactive substances, for example, proteins and peptides. Since the microbiome is a complex ecosystem with far-reaching effects on the metabolism of the host in the human intestine, it is examined not only on the genetic, but also on the proteomic and metabolic levels.[23]

With birth the development of the microbiome begins

In children who are born vaginally, the basic equipment of the microbiome is obtained automatically from the mother. This is not the case though for children who are delivered by Caesarean section. Of course, the bowel will eventually be colonized by bacteria, but it undergoes this process differently and later. It is quite important for the function of the immune system that its development is established as early as possible. Vaginal-born people in later life are in general healthier while allergies, asthma, autoimmune disease, obesity and even autism are found significantly more often in children who were born by Caesarean section.[24]

Diet is just as important to a child in the early years as love and care. Whether one is more susceptible to certain diseases or not is decided to a large extent in this period and is dependent on a functional microbiome. Later influence is possible, but it is better that it is established right from the start.

The Nestlé Research Center in Lausanne collaborated with Epigen Consortium in a study of factors that influence the development of intestinal bacteria in infants. The intestinal bacteria of infants aged three months and twelve months were studied and in February 2015, the research results were published. It was shown that infants who at the age of three months possessed a low diversity of gut bacteria, at the age of twelve months had a greater sensitivity to certain foods such as eggs, milk and peanuts than did those with a wider variety of intestinal bacteria.

The researchers found that two types of bacteria played a special role, namely enterobacteriaceae and bacteroidaceae. Infants who developed a sensitivity to certain foods by the age of twelve months, had different levels of these bacteria in the gut, compared with children without this sensitivity. The team used the results of a DNA analysis to analyze the bacteria from the stool of infants aged three months and twelve months respectively. The scientists were able to make predictions based on the bacteria that already existed within three months, about the development of food sensitivity in children aged up to one year.[25]

The researchers suggest that the microbiome is involved in the transfer of early life experiences to later life and health. However, the mechanisms for this are not yet known. To use the pattern of intestinal bacteria during childhood as a biomarker for future diseases, more research is needed. The scientists want to find out whether children with deviations from normal intestinal bacteria composition will develop food or other allergies. Thus, new routes could be found to prevent and treat allergies, possibly through the modification of the intestinal bacteria. First, an enlargement of the sample size and a new analysis of children aged between three to five years are planned.[26]

Living a long and healthy life as a research target

In the first 1,000 days, a special level of attention is paid in order to lay the foundation for a lifetime of good health or improvement this also applies, due to a demographic change, to the last stage in the life of a human being. This stage of life is by similar attention often severely compromised for people by neurodegenerative diseases and changes in the musculoskeletal system.

As life expectancy continues to increase, the age-related loss of muscle mass (sarcopenia) is becoming more common. The loss of muscle mass in old age is still underestimated on the medical side and not seen as an illness but as a normal part of the aging process. Thus recommendations to those it concerns are generally limited to performing strength training and taking proteins and multivitamins.

Age-related muscle loss can already begin from 50 years of age and by the age of 70, this process accelerates. The loss of muscle strength may then be about three percent annually. Depending on their way of life the elderly are affected to varying degrees by sarcopenia. However, no one, according to current knowledge, is immune from this.

Precisely because of the demographic development of an ever-increasing population of elderly people it is expected that sarcopenia in industrialized countries will become an increasing problem in the context of the economic consequences of public health. Therefore, in March 2015, the NIHS together with the Epigen Consortium launched a study to identify the molecular markers of sarcopenia.

This MEMOSA project (Multi-Ethnic Molecular Determinants of Human Sarcopenia) will help to identify the start of muscle loss in the elderly. The project aims to develop innovative nutritional solutions to counteract the problem. Sufferers could be thus be protected both against accidents, which are a consequence of muscle breakdown, and against early and prolonged bed rest. The nutritional treatment of sarcopenia is therefore a major contribution to improving the quality of life in old age.[27]

Numerous studies have shown that there are connections between cognitive decline in the elderly and factors such as diet, health of the heart and personal fitness. A new study named FINGER (Finnish Geriatric Intervention Study to Prevent Cognitive Impairment and Disability) has found that it is possible, if focus is given to these factors in the context of an intensive program, to prevent cognitive decline and thus avoid dementia.[28]

Dementia has many causes, and we now know that diet can influence the development and course of the disease. Various studies show that poor diet, as is often found in the elderly, increases the probability of the occurrence of age-related diseases.[29]

The current research aims to advance scientific understanding of Alzheimer's disease and other dementias, and the effects and the therapeutic potential of nutrition. Thus, for example, it has been demonstrated that a reduced glucose metabolism in the brain of an Alzheimer's patient plays an important role. This is one of the areas in which specific nutritional solutions can play a crucial role. Under the mantle of the Alzheimer's Association International Society to Advance Alzheimer's Research and Treatment a new PIA (Professional Interest Area) "Nutrition, Metabolism and Dementia" was established in which scientists, including those from the NIHS, and clinicians are working together to seek such solutions.

Already in 2013, scientists from the Nestlé Research Center and the Nestlé Institute of Health Sciences in collaboration with researchers from the University of Bologna, Italy, managed to discover the metabolic phenotype of healthy human aging and longevity. The study involved some 396 volunteers from northern Italy. They were divided into three age groups. The centenarians with an average age of 101 years were introduced because their physical and cognitive health made them practically ideal as examples of healthy aging. The second group of seniors had an average age of 70 years and the third group consisted of young adults with an average age of 31 years. The group of centenarians was again divided according to whether their parents were already particularly long-lived or not.[30]

Blood and urine samples of the study participants were analyzed to establish a metabolomic approach regarding the characteristics of the aging process. Analysis of blood samples revealed that certain lipids were clearly changed in the centenarians. Other substances were also found which had a remarkable resemblance to those of the group of younger participants. Between the centenarians whose parents had already reached an advanced age, and those where that was not the case, there was a significant difference in the metabolic phenotype.

In general it was found that the centenarians were significantly better at responding to oxidative and chronic inflammatory conditions, which is an indication of the causes of longevity. In the centenarians a complex metabolic conversion had obviously taken place in which the microbiome participated. This metabolic conversion led to a balance between inflammatory and anti-inflammatory processes.

The researchers now have the physiological markers that indicate a long life of good health. However, this knowledge is not sufficient and must be deepened by further studies with other populations and other genetic backgrounds material. To this end, populations in various parts of Europe are being studied to determine to what extent the diet of the Italian participants might influence their metabolic signature. The goal of achieving through diet and lifestyle a long life lived in good health has come significantly closer because of this study.

CHAPTER 5:
THE RESPONSIBILITY OF THE FOOD INDUSTRY

The path from nutrition research to finished product takes place in three major steps. Discovering, developing, introducing. Elsewhere one speaks of the 3-D principle: discover, develop and deploy. Not every piece of new scientific knowledge that is gained in basic research is likely to be implemented immediately in a new or improved product. It is the task of the various business units to decide which findings and discoveries are to be developed further and in what way.

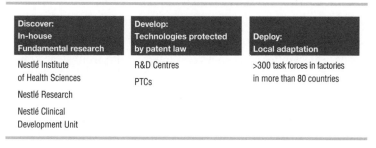

Discover: In-house Fundamental research	Develop: Technologies protected by patent law	Deploy: Local adaptation
Nestlé Institute of Health Sciences	R&D Centres	>300 task forces in factories in more than 80 countries
Nestlé Research	PTCs	
Nestlé Clinical Development Unit		

Fig. 5: We have unmatched abilities for innovation at our disposal

The consumer is the focus from the very beginning

Until the finished product is created, it is often a long and winding road, which all participants must travel together in a company. What has been found effective in laboratory tests and in studies, is far from the finished product which can convince and delight the consumer. The further steps in the development of new products revolve around what is known worldwide as "design thinking".

This involves developing ideas that are put into prototypes and their function tested, in order to draw conclusions about how you can still improve the ideas and develop new prototypes, which will then be tested again under practical conditions. If you arrive, during this iterative process, at a point that meets the expectations of a future product, it goes into the next phase which is to develop the necessary industrial manufacturing process. If this phase has been successfully mastered, you can begin to introduce the new product on a trial basis in a market which has sufficient potential for interested parties.[1]

The success of this test phase depends on there being nothing to prevent the opening up of further markets. The development of product ideas and the concept of value for the consumer are certainly the key points to encourage consumers to try the product and then to continue to use it. In fact, of five or maybe even ten new products only one is as successful as was expected. One must of course also take into account that consumers in different markets have different needs, expect different services and interpret the promise of a given product differently.

In the past 60 years, it was often enough to offer consumers a new or improved product that was recognizable enough to convince them to purchase the product. Today it has become more important, not only to understand the behavior of consumers, but also the underlying basis of the decision.

Of course, all the major food manufacturers conduct research in the field of Health and Wellness. In the field of science, the food industry is in the view of the Fraunhofer Institute expected to provide the following services:

Improved simulation of physiological processes and biological systems for research on diet. This includes the development of new methods for the quantification of food consumption and nutrient intake and the development of new methods for the determination of bioavailability and the metabolic fate of food ingredients. Overall, the exchange of knowledge between research in the corporate and public sectors such as universities and other research institutions should be improved. Within the Fraunhofer study the activities of Nestlé Research were cited as an example to be adopted worldwide.

The growing market for specialty and wellness food

In terms of nutrition, we are facing a "reset" mode because there is a whole new attitude to health within health-oriented personalization and resource conservation.

Putting this in perspective: Euromonitor estimates the global size for "Health and Wellness" fortified food in 2016 at USD 165 bn. Similary, the Transparency Market Research establishes the current global nutraceuticals market at USD 180 bn and forecasts it to reach USD 280 bn by the end of 2021. The global nutraceuticals market goes significantly beyond Health Science products as it comprises the functional food and beverages, dietary supplements and also personal care and pharmaceuticals products. Taking an even broader definition, Euromonitor estimates a total world market for specialty and wellness food of currently over Swiss Francs 700 bn a year, with growth for the next years of nine percent annually.[2] As with other markets that did not exist before, forecasts for health-oriented personalization of food require vision, rather than sophisticated statistical methods. It reminds me of a story told by former colleagues from Nokia: in an early phase, the global market for mobile phones was expected to be saturated once reaching 500,000 devices.

The idea of a "Nutrition, Health and Wellness Company"

Back in 2000, I thought about the possibility of Nestlé moving from being a pure food manufacturer to a Wellbeing Company. The basis and, as it were the door opener, for Wellbeing is a balanced, healthy diet for the different stages of life and lifestyles. Wellbeing includes but is more than the physical condition and emotional range of well-being, extending to appearance and the desire for an active and long, healthy life.

A Wellbeing Company would be based on three pillars, a Food Company, a pharmaceutical company and a cosmetic and personal care company, thereby creating a new industry. My Board then decided to dispense with the pharmaceutical company aspect because the business model is completely different from that of a company in the consumer goods industry; but it gave its consent to create, in the long term, a strategie goal of becoming "Nutrition, Health and Wellness Company".

It was already clear that in the long term the aim was to achieve a personalized diet and personalized health prevention. To establish this, we needed an improved diagnostics, but not a private pharmaceutical company. The science of personalized health nutrition is about finding efficient and cost effective ways to prevent and treat the acute and chronic diseases of the 21st century.

This reorientation led the company closer to the pharmaceutical industry, but it retained its focus on the consumer within the broad consumer goods industry as a holistic objective at the core of its activities. While in the food industry the individual consumer is crucial, namely whether they buy a product or not, in the pharmaceutical industry the emphasis is not on consumers, but whether a drug works or not. Nestlé has the great advantage that it has always been focused on the consumer.

That Nestlé repositioned itself as a health company, was not primarily an ethical decision but a business one. I was convinced that in the next 20 years the subject of health would drive the next wave of innovation in the food industry. While convenience has been the value engine in the past 40 years, in the next 20 years the great value of products will be judged on the basis of their health benefits. An important prerequisite for this repositioning as a "Nutrition, Health and Wellness Company" was a reorientation of research and development activities.

HealthCare Nutrition—Nutritional solutions for people with specific medical conditions

The foundations for the future of a new industry were already laid in 1986, when Nestlé went into the HealthCare Nutrition business, which was initially an integral part of Nestlé Nutrition. This area was expanded. They offered food supplements for the sick and elderly, and also developed a screening tool that recognized the existing threat of malnutrition. There were also products for people with cancer and gastrointestinal disorders, and for enteral nutrition through feeding tubes.

With the acquisition of Novartis Medical Nutrition division mid 2007, Nestlé took a great step forward in the global market for medical nutrition achieving second place behind the US pharmaceutical company Abbott. The field of infant nutrition overseen by Nestlé Nutrition has been strengthened by the acquisition of the Gerber baby foods business from Novartis in 2007. Nestlé became the worldwide leader in nutritional solutions.

Nestlé Health Science Company—a new health frontier arises

In 2011, the newly created Nestlé Health Science company (NHSc) became operational. Along with the simultaneously founded Nestlé Institute of Health Sciences (NIHS) these have the task of developing science-based personalized health products. The portfolio is aimed at important challenges in our society: healthy aging, brain health, gastrointestinal health and inborn errors of metabolism. The

NHSc should from the outset shape and advance the role of nutritional therapies in health management.

The Nestlé Health Science company's goal is to become the world leader of science-based, nutritional therapies. It is divided into three divisions, Consumer Care, Medical Nutrition and Novel Therapeutic Nutrition. The starting point was HealthCare Nutrition, which was part of Nestlé Nutrition and today forms the core activities of Nestlé Health Science. NHSc is a health-science company engaged in advancing the role of nutritional therapy to change the course of health for consumers, patients and our partners in healthcare. Its portfolio of nutrition solutions, diagnostics, devices and drugs, targets a number of health areas, such as inborn errors of metabolism, pediatric and acute care, obesity care, healthy aging as well as gastrointestinal and brain health. Through investing in innovation and leveraging leading edge science, we bring forward innovative nutritional therapies with proven clinical, health economic value and quality of life benefits.

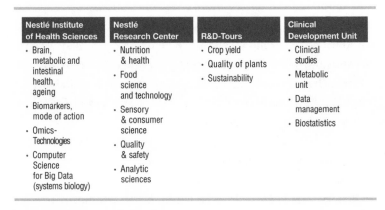

Nestlé Institute of Health Sciences	Nestlé Research Center	R&D-Tours	Clinical Development Unit
• Brain, metabolic and intestinal health, ageing • Biomarkers, mode of action • Omics-Technologies • Computer Science for Big Data (systems biology)	• Nutrition & health • Food science and technology • Sensory & consumer science • Quality & safety • Analytic sciences	• Crop yield • Quality of plants • Sustainability	• Clinical studies • Metabolic unit • Data management • Biostatistics

Fig. 6: Four fundamental research axes

In Consumer Care we offer a range of nutritional solutions (Boost in North America, Meritene in Europe) for general health concerns or specific health conditions following self-diagnosis or guidance from healthcare professionals. Through retail and pharmacy channels these nutritional solutions are directly accessible to consumers and available without a prescription. It's a fast growing area as people are increasingly health aware, with access to the knowledge about nutritional needs related to healthy and active ageing.

Our Medical Nutrition range covers specific dietary needs of patients suffering from illnesses or specific disease states. We are addressing nutritional needs associated with a number of categories; Inborn Errors of Metabolism, Pediatric Care & food allergy, Acute Care (including critically ill, swallowing disorders and cancer), as well as Metabolic, Obesity and Cancer Care. Our Medical Nutrition products are recommended by healthcare professional and used in hospitals, nursing homes, and in home care.

In Novel Therapeutic Nutrition we are investing in companies with a range of nutrient-based technology platforms aiming to bring forward clinically proven innovations, initially in the areas of brain and gastrointestinal health.

For instance in gastrointestinal health, one of our initiatives is to invest in the development of microbiome therapeutics. These have the potential to address the underlying causes of many types of diseases by restoring the gut microbiota to a healthy state. This healthy state can be disrupted by different health conditions such as trauma or even drugs. The company has a strong product pipeline, which currently includes more than 40 promising projects. In New Jersey, in the United States, a new Nestlé Product Technology Centre has been established with the task of driving innovation in the three priority areas of Nestlé Health Science.

Cooperation and takeovers strengthen the scientific foundations

More than 5,000 scientists and researchers around the world work for Nestlé. Its cooperation with leading experts in the respective fields in universities and biotech companies multiplies this potential. Through acquisitions and joint ventures the results of cutting-edge research in health and nutritional science are made available. As early as 2010 Vitaflo was acquired, a company based in Liverpool, UK, which develops nutritional solutions for people with genetically inherited, metabolic diseases that are diagnosed shortly after birth.

In 2011, Prometheus Laboratories, based in San Diego, California, was acquired. The company specializes in innovative diagnostic and pharmaceutical products in the field of gastrointestinal diseases and cancer. The integration of diagnostic and pharmaceutical products allows Nestlé Health Science to offer physicians more targeted approaches to treatment optimization.

The acquisition of Pamlab in 2013 enhanced the therapeutic areas of brain health and metabolic health. The American company has an innovative portfolio of medical food products for patients with mild cognitive impairment depression and diabetes-related neuropathy.

A minority stake has also existed since 2012 in Accera, USA. Accera specialized in the research, development and commercialization of medical nutrition for neurodegenerative diseases such as Alzheimer's disease. This participation with Accera enables Nestlé Health Science to broaden its portfolio in the field of brain health.

In 2012, NHSc and Chi-Med, a Chinese pharmaceutical company, formed a 50/50 joint venture under the name of Nutrition Science Partners Limited (NSP). NSP develops innovative nutritional and medicinal products derived from botanical plants. First, the focus is on gastrointestinal health, and later on metabolic health and brain health. With this joint venture NSP has access to the extensive botanical library of Chi-Med, one of the world's leading libraries of traditional Chinese medicine. This lists over 1,200 different medicinal plants and more than 50,000 plant extracts.

In January 2015, NHSc invested 65 million dollars in Seres Therapeutics Inc, headquartered in Cambridge, Massachusetts. Seres is the world leader in developing microbiome therapeutics (Ecobiotics). In January 2016, NHSc signed an exclusive agreement with Seres in the areas of Clostridium difficile infections and of Inflammatory Bowel Disease. Another investment was made in Lipid therapeutics, a German company developing novel therapies for the treatment of ulcerative colitis.

In addition to investing in Seres, Nestlé Health Science signed in a strategic innovation partnership with Flagship Ventures, based in Cambridge, Mass. Flagship Ventures is a leading company for the establishment and financing of venture capital companies focused on innovation in health care and sustainability. Together, start-up companies are supported that work on healthy diets and therapies. Nestlé Health Science thus has early access to innovative knowledge and technology through Flagship, which can then be exploited by minority direct investment, licensing, joint ventures or acquisitions.

Nestle Skin Health for the health of skin, hair and nails

Another company that deals with health products on a scientific basis, is Nestlé Skin Health S.A. With its establishment in June 2014 Nestlé expanded its business activities to the field of specialized medical skin care products. A new company, Galderma, was founded as a 50/50 joint venture with L'Oréal, which already held a leading position in the industry. With the complete acquisition of Galderma and the creation of Nestlé Skin Health a global leader has been created that focuses on meeting the world's increasing demand in the region of skin health with a wide range of innovative and scientifically proven products. Bübchen, the existing Nestlé business with skincare products for babies, has been integrated into the new unit.

Nestle Skin Health aims to improve the quality of life through science-based solutions for the health of skin, hair and nails. The skin is one of the most important human organs. It protects us from harmful environmental influences, serving as a cover for our bodies and affects our behavior, our outward appearance, our self-image and wellbeing. With a growing life expectancy our needs and expectations furthermore change with respect to the skin. We also want to look well-aged, feel comfortable and take an active role in society.

The products and solutions of Nestle Skin Health protect and nourish the skin, improve their health, alleviate and heal skin damage and help restore a healthy skin image. Today about 3,000 skin diseases are known, more than for any other organ in our body. Galderma is the Medical Solutions division of Nestle Skin Health. Working closely with health experts, the company determines the requirements of patients in order to develop effective solutions.

Today, we observe a significant shift in the general understanding of wellbeing. This trend drives a strong growth in the Aesthetic Medicine segment. Galderma's portfolio includes medical products for minimally invasive and non-invasive methods for restoring and beautifying the skin's image, performed by qualified health professionals.

The newly created division of Consumer Skin Health uses the consumer knowledge and scientific expertise of the company to make leading consumer brands such as our skincare assortment Cetaphil and our sunscreen series Daylong that are science-based innovations brought to a wider market.

By 2020 over a billion people will be over 60 years old worldwide. Thus, not only health needs but also the needs of healthcare professionals and their roles change. Nestle Skin Health therefore has launched a number of important initiatives which should contribute to research, training and development of solutions for lifelong health.

Growth expectations for Nestlé Skin Health is in double digits, while for Nestlé Health Science it is in the higher single digits. Overall, therefore, Nestlé is well on the way to becoming a company that is built on the three pillars of nutrition, health and wellness.

A look at the evolution of consumer behavior in recent years by the Fraunhofer Institute shows that growth will be achieved in the food sector and nutrition particularly in the areas of "health", "enjoyment" and "convenience." New profitable and fast-growing market segments, however, have almost exclusively been established by big business here. Small and medium enterprises, at least by 2010, lacked their own research and development activities in order to generate real innovations. That has still not changed.[3]

Nutrition as therapy

The pharmaceutical industry will in the future continue to focus on developing drugs that can cure diseases and that can be used under the supervision of physicians to improve health. To exclude side effects or to reduce them and to find the right dosage, costly clinical trials will be necessary in the future. The research involved is expensive and lengthy.

Within the healthcare industry there is another area, the non-prescription, homeopathic and natural remedies found in vitamins and dietary supplements. It is likely that this is an approach that the new area of the Health and Wellness industry will adopt or already has.

The conventional food industry will continue to offer products that provide the human body with nutrients but also products that can be enriched with essential micronutrients and trace elements. By contrast, the Health and Wellness industry has on the one hand initially focused on understanding the functioning of the human body to the molecular level. It studies the active substances in daily food down to the molecular basis. Through this complex scientific discovery process fundamentally new nutriceuticals will be developed, i.e. foods that are suitable for the treatment or prevention of diseases.

Competition for a longer life

However, it is not just the major food manufacturers who conduct research in the area of Health and Wellness. There are also initiatives from the financially strong IT industry. For instance, Google founded the biotechnology company Calico in 2013. The name stands for California Life Company, and their goal is to develop methods to combat age-related diseases. They also aim to find out how to prolong life.[4]

In 2012, the market for so-called regenerative medicine was estimated at over 2.6 billion US dollars and it is projected that by 2019 the market volume will triple. But such research is not just about the prolongation of life in itself, but, as with Nestlé, also that human life will be made up of more healthy years and will mean a better quality of life.[5]

Calico, like all start-up companies in Silicon Valley, has ambitious goals, which go far beyond what we consider today to be realistic. It is hoped, for instance, to find solutions that will extend the life span of people by several decades. If that were to be made possible, first, one would have to beat cancer, which itself decreases the average life expectancy on average by three years. One can see quite clearly how far the objectives of Calico are from what seems feasible and what is sought by Nestlé.

It is still not clear how and why people age. Is it because the DNA in our cells throughout life experiences so much damage that the repair mechanisms no longer work and cause this damage in the end to lead to sickness and death? Is it diminishing mitochondrial function? Is it loss of stem cells? Does the decoding of the human proteome help or is it important to advance the exploration of the microbiome? Likely a holistic approach is necessary requiring a broad-based system approach to research.

Solutions for certain life situations and risk groups

It is not just in the first 1,000 days of one's life that proper nutrition plays an important role, but also in old age. An elderly person with osteoporosis needs larger amounts of calcium and vitamin D. In this case, a dietary supplement with supplements is certainly useful.

Many older people are severely limited by dysphagia, and one of the possible causes is that they can no longer break down the food properly and transport it to the stomach. It comes down to making the right nutrients available, and that is best achieved with a liquid food which has the proper viscosity and is enriched accordingly. The difference from the pharmaceutical industry is that in relation to such products the food industry not only provides the ingredients, but also the know-how to make this food taste good, have a consistent appearance and be prepared in a manner that those affected will also enjoy eating it.[6]

Physical exercise boosts your metabolism. People who have difficulties being active because their age, illness or disability prevents them from taking part in sports, need additional support. Scientists from Nestlé have found a way to enhance the effect of exercise on the body through an appropriate diet. The discovery of a nutrition solution that mimics the newly discovered mechanism of action of the drug C13 can promote the fat burning effect of sport on the human metabolism. Instead of a strenuous exercise program, people with natural drug mimetics may be able to boost their metabolism even with moderate exercise. Without having to exert themselves but by regulating the energy management of the body better it may help the elderly and the sick to stay fit.[7]

Poor nutrition makes one aggressive

Bernard Gesch, a scientist from the University of Oxford, discovered that the occupants of many British prisons remained extremely violent. He therefore organized an experiment in several prisons, through which he sought to test whether prisoners became more peaceful when they ate better. Studies had previously shown that prisoners usually have a very monotonous diet, which consists primarily of white bread, French fries and sweets. But when offered a diet rich in vitamins and minerals such as fruits, vegetables and salad, they refrained from eating it.[8]

In the experiment, Gesch gave the prisoners, in addition to the normal prison diet, a tablet containing unsaturated fatty acids, minerals and vitamins. After four and a half months, he came to the conclusion that the prisoners who took these tablets were involved on average in 37 percent fewer acts of violence and other serious incidents than those prisoners who received only standard food. Obviously the diet has a direct link to behavioral problems. If further experiments confirm these results, they will certainly have an impact not only on improving prison meals, but also on the nutritional concepts used in kindergartens, schools, hospitals, old people's homes and businesses, as well as in the military.

Food for extreme situations

In March 2015, the solar plane "Solar Impulse 2" was launched from Abu Dhabi into the Earth's orbit. In July 2015, it achieved a record by flying for almost 8300 km from Japan to Hawaii in 118 hours. At times during this long flight they were barely able to move, yet, they had to stay mentally fit.

One of the biggest challenges was to provide the pilots with all the essential nutrients needed at an altitude of 8,000 meters in a non-pressurized cabin. Both the food and its packaging had to be optimized to withstand extreme temperatures, yet be easy to eat and taste good.

At high altitudes, people often lose their appetite. Therefore, two different types of food were designed, one for consumption higher than 3,500 meters and one for lower levels. In developing the food the individual nutritional profiles of the pilots were analyzed, so that they could be fed adequately during the 35,000 km journey, which was divided into twelve flights and during which they were exposed to 500 hours in the air at extreme loads of pressure. The data collected as part of this research are now being used to develop more foods for extreme situations.[9]

CHAPTER 6:
THE RESPONSIBILITY OF POLICY

This chapter is about three policy areas that are related to each other not only at a national but also at an international level. It involves the links between social and health policy, development policy and competition policy. Social systems and health systems will in the future be increasingly dominated by the need to change existing conditions to avoid possible future diseases. Instead of "diagnosis and treatment" the emphasis will be on "prediction and prevention", as the prevention of diseases is the key to a strong economy.

Through prevention, each individual has an improved quality of life and the chance for a long, healthy life. Prevention must be considered by those who are healthy as well as those who are already suffering from a chronic disease with a view to avoiding further complications. When considering the cost of disease prevention clearly ethical reasons come first. As such, it is unethical and thus unjustified to engage in a discussion of who counts or not in terms of the costs of extending lives.

If we start from the premise of an aging population, the working capacity must be extended, and that will only possible through appropriate preventive measures. In this case there is not only a responsibility for providers of health and pension insurance but also the employers, who have a vested interest in seeing a fall in the incidence of ill health amongst an aging workforce.

In the long term, medical costs in an economy can be effectively reduced through efficient health care. For this, it is necessary, however, to identify all the appropriate preventive measures. When appropriate prevention measures are effective, they are able to contribute to an improvement in health care financing. Prevention is to be carried out on three levels.

Primary prevention will focus on healthy people, who do not have symptoms of disease or who are in a position to be able to control their behavior so as to eliminate any symptoms or postpone these to a later date. This health care is aimed at a broad population and is already in use in kindergartens and schools. Secondary prevention primarily includes screening tests for diagnosing diseases which are not yet visible at the symptom level, such as cancer screening. The third level of prevention is to avoid a worsening of symptoms or the occurrence of additional complications in established illnesses.

When it comes to changing the health behavior of individuals, state institutions mainly rely on the information of their citizens. They have the opportunity to take restrictive measures and intervene only on the basis of recommendations via bans, for example, on tobacco and alcohol, and other actions that impact the lives of citizens. Denmark experimented with such measures by instituting a fat tax, while the US is doing so with a ban on artificial transfats in food, to be implemented in 2018. But such interventions for most health officials do not seem to be first choice solutions as this tends to have disruptive effects on the entire economy.

At present it is not yet common in most health systems for physicians to be sufficiently rewarded for increasing the preparedness and responsiveness of their patients. It will therefore be necessary to consider these benefits in the medical fee catalogs accordingly. Since the level of health care is also in direct relation to the level of education of citizens, the education systems will have to strengthen their role in helping health literacy of the population. In addition, the internet provides an increasingly important channel to inform people about these issues.

Today, in most countries, the problem is to adequately target groups for preventive measures, mainly people with a high risk of disease, and, in general, to define and develop optimal approaches for these target populations. There is still uncertainty as to what programs are actually suitable for health care and how the financing is to take place. As such, all political powers will be required to work on solutions. The sooner this happens the better.

The ideal solution of individualized, science-based health care is still far off. Realizing this will require comprehensive scientific and technological developments, the achievement of cost effectiveness, widespread availability and the ability to apply any solutions on a large scale. The road to individualized precision medicine is long. In the first instance, focus will need to be given to improving scientific and technical methods for identifying target populations and addressing them specifically. In this context, we now speak of a stratified medicine, i.e. a medicine that is aimed at certain groups, or strata.

Another important aspect when considering precautionary health systems is the ability to influence risk factors. We still believe that these risk factors are mainly in the domain of each individual's influence. However, it must be seen whether a "behavioral prevention" is sufficient or not with regard to larger populations or whether changes in peoples' living conditions ("situational prevention") is just as or even more necessary. This means, however, that external risk factors, such as emissions from motor vehicle traffic or by urbanization and other environmental factors, such as an increase in UV radiation, must be considered.

Preventive health systems as part of global health

Preventive health care systems are an essential element of global health. The global convergence of living and consumption habits is accompanied by the spread of non-communicable chronic diseases, which are not only a problem of developed countries, but also increasingly occur in emerging and developing countries. Today, we are not only seeing the challenge of preventable deaths from infection diseases, but we are seeing non-communicable diseases threaten development opportunities, economic growth and the entire social and political stability of a whole region.

All forms of disease in the emerging and developing countries are a major cause of poverty and inequality as well as associated conflicts. The consequences of climate change in these countries are an additional public health challenge. A permanent challenge is still the fight against hunger and malnutrition. According to the WHO Constitution, health is a state of complete physical, mental and social wellbeing and not merely the absence of disease or infirmity. In this context, human rights are of particular importance to food.

Overall, it is clear that global health issues are closely related to many other policies, such as development, trade, industry, food, agriculture, research, education and environmental protection. Global health issues are thus no longer treated exclusively by health experts but by a large number of governmental, intergovernmental and non-state actors.

This "international health" has traditionally been focused on developing countries and their health problems, that is, on infectious diseases, water problems, sanitary conditions and malnutrition. Meanwhile, the term "international health" was replaced with the new concept of "global health". This term includes, alongside existing priorities, an emphasis on prevention and on a common understanding of health as a public good that requires the cooperation of all stakeholders and places the importance of systems and structures in the foreground.

Especially in developing countries, the context of globalization and urbanization created a double burden of classic health risks from communicable diseases and lifestyle diseases. The goal of Global Health is to enable people to gain more control over their health. This requires the joint efforts of international organizations, national government agencies and civil society and the private sector. To establish a workable relationship between government and business, both a national and international competition policy is necessary to keep everyone involved.

Ensuring fair competition as a political task

With regard to the policies of national governments and international organizations my view, similar to that held by Nestlé, has long been one based on ordoliberalism, a German variety of social liberalism. This thinking implies that states have the task of creating the conditions for free competition in the economic sphere, and keeping it operational, in order to ensure individual freedom. Regulated competition prevents the emergence of private sector market power and establishes a legal framework within which the players can act.

According to theories of ordoliberalism, a State's objectives can be realized when it recognizes the following principles in its economic system:

- securing free market prices and a functioning price mechanism;
- ensuring open markets or preventing market entry barriers;
- freedom of contract;
- equality before the law;
- private ownership of means of production and
- ensuring that private-sector decision-making power and responsibility correspond to the polluter pays principle.

In addition, the state should be able to make timely interventions in economic activity, while ensuring that these are not detrimental to the market price mechanism. Indeed, globalization needs a frameword.

For its part, Nestlé applies the above approach in all nation states where it has factories and behaves accordingly towards all local consumers, employees and state institutions. Companies are essential parts of the social structure of each country. They mus therefore meet certain obligations in respect to the environment in which they operate and cannot ignore or disregard these.

In addition, a global expert also needs clear and inviolable principles and values on issues such as the quality and safety of products, ways of dealing with the various stakeholders, environmental and ecological conditions and human rights.

With these principles, Nestlé contributes to the increased prosperity of the countries that have given the company a home. And it does this not just by bringing good products to market, or bringing expertise and new technologies, or paying wages and buying raw materials. An international company also ensures above all more competition. It forces suppliers, commercial and financial partners and authorities to improve their own practices.

When people no longer have to fight to avoid hunger, new values are created alongside more prosperity, more education and a higher degree of awareness of these values. That is also a good basis for the development of democracy. And with more democracy, greater attention and respect is secured for human rights. This requires more than the declaration of values; it requires specific actions.

The long-term success of a company is only possible, in my opinion, when its activities, principles and practices, find general agreement among all parties, be they owners, consumers, civil society, employees or authorities. For this reason it is in the long-term interests of each manager, to conscientiously abide by laws, to develop an understanding of social issues and to ensure that the company's activities and the interests of the society in which it operates go hand in hand. This naturally requires the involvement of stakeholders to strengthen dialogue and deepen understanding of important social issues.

CHAPTER 7:
THE RESPONSIBILITY OF EACH INDIVIDUAL

Everyone, regardless of origin and social status, is entitled to a standard of living which guarantees him and his family health and well-being, and this includes food and medical care. This is laid down in Article 25 of the United Nations' 1948 Universal Declaration of Human Rights. It is certainly an individual's personal responsibility to do everything that is possible to meet this requirement. But often enough one's strength, knowledge and skills do not matter if natural and social conditions preclude the realization of this ideal. In such a case a person is dependent on the assistance of other people and institutions that can help.

What can we decide and what not?

The life sciences have hitherto assumed that our diet and food preferences are based on complex interactions between the genetic makeup of a person, their environment and social environment and on cultural components. Most people think they know how to eat properly and healthily. However, the vast majority do not follow their own ideas. Why is there such a difference between what a person considers desirable, and what they actually do?

Individual psychology makes inherited traits and personality structures acquired through socialization and education responsible for this discrepancy between thought and action. There is seen to be a failure of willpower, discipline, self-control and rational insight. Social psychology sees the causes as being rooted in the social environment of the individual and the complicity of social influences, especially advertising. For neuroscientists, the reasons people do not act according to their own intelligence lies in unconscious processes of the brain that are beyond conscious control.

Three evolutionary biologists have now submitted a further explanation of our eating habits. Joe Alcock, Carlo C. Maley and C. Athena Aktipis evaluated 120 scientific publications in order to answer the question whether our eating behavior is influenced by gastrointestinal microbes.[1]

Not all decisions are made in the head

The fight against the craving for sugar and fatty meals is one fought by many people every day. People know that unhealthy food is a major cause of health problems. This is true not only in relation to obesity, diabetes and cardiovascular disease, but also to cancers of the stomach and the intestinal tract, and even to sleep, which leads to decreased physical and mental performance. Nevertheless, unhealthy eating patterns are difficult to change.

Therefore, the researchers have suggested a very different approach to lack of control exhibited over appetite: they may have found a conflict of interest between the needs of the intestinal bacteria of a person and their eating habits in the course of evolution. As a result of this conflict, microbes manipulate the behavior of people in order to ensure their own wellbeing, even if it harms human health.

Basically, we're leaving out the fact that our microbiome performs important functions in the human body, by being involved in food utilization and the development of the immune system. However, not all microbes have similar interests but are instead in a competition for habitat and nutrients. A differentiated intestine population is therefore likely to be too busy keeping each other in check to get enough energy and other resources and to defend itself, as is the case in a microbiome, which has a significantly lower bacterial diversity.

The larger the group of certain microbes, the better the opportunities to manipulate their human host and satisfy their own needs. Hence the hypothesis is that a less diversified microbiome goes along with unhealthy lifestyles and a greater degree of obesity.

There are now numerous results that may scientifically prove that a person can be manipulated by their microbiome. Some strains of bacteria thrive best when they receive carbohydrates, while others prefer whole grains and some fats. In Japanese microbes it has even been discovered that they have become specialized in the digestion of algae, which are indeed an integral part of Japanese cuisine. In African children who were fed sorghum, microbes could be found that could use this specific cellulose.

The same microbes that are "omnivores" maintain an ongoing fight for survival in the human gut. To win this battle, they have to manipulate their hosts as much as possible to suit their needs. Thus, it has been found that the microbiome is composed differently in people who are addicted to chocolate than in humans where chocolate consumption is not particularly important.[2] But whether the microbiome affects chocolate consumption or vice versa, is not yet clear.

Through experiments conducted on mice, it has been shown that there is a connection between behavior and the composition of the microbiome. Here especially the central nervous system plays a major role. When babies cry because they are hungry, then their discomfort may well be inspired by their microbiome. It is not the child that feels a lack of nutrients, but its microbiome. By way of discomfort, and as in adults, the microbes signal when they lack food. It is hypothesized that the bacteria can control relevant neurons specifically to emit pain signals. But these are by no means all the instruments available to the microbes to manipulate people.[3]

In a study of aseptic Bubble mice, it was found that they have different taste receptors for fat on the tongue and in the intestine than mice with a normal microbiome. Another study showed that Bubble mice that strongly prefer sweet food have a greater number of sweetness receptors populating their microbiome than others. Clearly, the microbes are able to transform the food preferences of their hosts by a transformation of the taste receptors, or by a change in the perception of these receptors. This can then also control the level of satiety of the hosts.[4]

It is known that the vagus nerve regulates feeding behavior and body weight. It thus becomes obvious that the intestinal microbes affect the activity of the vagus nerve using neurochemicals, with the result that a person eats more than they would otherwise have done. More than 50 percent of the mood hormones dopamine and serotonin are formed in mammals by the intestines and they are thus acted upon by some of the intestinal inhabitants. Thus the production of hormones that stimulate the appetite is a very easy way for the microbiome to manipulate people. Who then actually controls the appetite and feeling of hunger by individuals remains an open question.[5]

The desire to eat a lot does not arise when little food is available or one is fasting. The opposite is the case. The more energy is absorbed, and the more one-sided the diet, the greater the desire to eat more. This is probably because the composition of the microbiome is changed unilaterally because of the food supply. Once the unfavorable microbes have managed to gain the upper hand a person will no longer be able to control his eating behavior.

Researchers even found evidence that obesity is contagious, not on a social level (such as by changing eating habits of specific groups), but rather as an infection by intestinal germs. It is now proven that the entire microbiome of a person can also be detected in its habitat, such as the apartment one lives in. This even applies to hotel rooms, which are colonized with new microbes within a few hours of new guests arriving. So when people have contact with each other, it is almost inevitable that intestinal bacteria are transmitted. If they are able to change the eating habits of their host, they can also do this in a new host.[6]

Food addiction incidentally differs considerably from addiction to drugs or alcohol. These require ever higher doses to achieve the desired effect in the consumer. As the microbes that control eating behavior are not addictive, but only want to satisfy their nutritional needs, a healthy person with a healthy appetite will not necessarily "overeat", unless there are other causes of disease. However, while there are certainly people who find pleasure in their gluttony, current studies suggest that drug abuse and gluttony are caused by different mechanisms.

Using probiotics can certainly change the composition and hence the operation of the microbiome in a person such that someone who consumes the same amount still loses weight. Namely, it is not the case that only microbes can manipulate the individual but the converse is also true. Through prebiotics, probiotics and antibiotics the composition of the microbiome can in time change. What matters is making this change permanent.[7]

The suspected manipulation of their own behavior by the microbiome can not be recognized by the individual, because it forms a community with its microbiome and it can not perceive the body separately. Food intake is not usually controlled rationally but by feelings and physical sensations. Since the causes can also arise from the microbiome, it is important that the different species be classified within the microbiome to describe their functions and so understand the relationships between them. That does not mean that in future one can exclude considering the circumstances of people to understand nutritional behavior.

Traditions, diet myths and ideological trends

Individual eating habits in Western societies are increasingly influenced by the social environment and increasingly less so by tradition. The only exceptions are diets that are motivated by religion and are regulated by a more or less large number of commandments or prohibitions.

In childhood, acquired food preferences and habits that are often maintained for a lifetime are attributed to the socialization process not the maintenance of traditions. Even so, across all societies, food and eating behavior have retained their signalling and messaging importance. Through what we eat, how we eat and where we eat, we share something about ourselves with others. Food and nutrition determine belonging and communicate what is important to us to the outside world.

Diet myths instead of knowledge

Concrete understanding about food production, and in particular the aspects of quality, are often replaced by vague romantic notions and by nutritional myths. In addition to criteria of taste, such as freshness, origin, naturalness (no preservatives and flavor enhancers), some consider regional specification as a critical variable to assess quality. Its significance is, however, questionable.

According to two-thirds of consumers, the biggest quality-related factor in food is its processing.[8] The transparency of the production chain and its sustainability are often unclear. How environmentally friendly a product is from the very beginning, how long and in what ways it was transported and whether social standards were adhered to in the production, is especially difficult for the consumer to assess if it is not a reliable brand.

The low level of consumer knowledge manifests itself today in fears about certain foods, something we have seen since 1961 when the American Heart Association published its studies on cholesterol.

In these studies, the Association blamed the increasing number of heart attacks and strokes on foods such as milk, butter, or beef. In her book, "The Big Fat Surprise: Why Butter, Meat and Cheese Belong in a Healthy Diet", the journalist Nina Teicholz, meanwhile demonstrates that the nutritional advice given in this case by government and consumer organizations was not based on sufficiently reliable scientific work.[9]

And so, for almost 50 years many Americans have given up red meat, cheese, milk and eggs or have only consumed them with a guilty conscience, without there being any evidence-based scientific studies to support such fears. Historian Warren J. Belasco called the resulting movement "Negative Nutrition".[10]

Back to nature—the yearning for the original

Subjective assessments, coupled with imprecise ideals, are the basis in many places for the concept of a healthy diet. This goes beyond the focus on a balanced and healthy diet and is an ideological position, which also includes the origin and production methods of food products.[11]

Consumers who eat a balanced diet and are healthy, place, at the same time, an above average value on fruits and vegetables that are offered seasonally, and on the welfare of animals that provide meat. The products should come from the local region and be produced naturally and without genetic engineering. These factors are ranked higher than the classification of organic products in the preference scale of consumers. These preferences for food production reflect a widespread longing for the original, which is characterized by clean nature, animal welfare and a life lived in line with the seasons. How far these ideals are realized and also how consistently is another matter.

Women are, on the whole, more concerned with nutrition than men, and tend far more than men to evaluate nutrition according to ideology. This is also reflected in the typology of eating habits.

The 2009 study "Nutrition in Germany" by Nestlé SA defined seven food types that are relevant today. These can be divided into three groups.[12]

Almost half of Germans are assigned, according to this study, to the health conscious group, which includes the diet types of "health idealists", "problem conscious" and "nest warmer." One third of the population belongs to the "short of time" group. There you will find the food types of "the harried" and the "modern multi-optional". The group titled "uninterested" has a share of 20 percent, consisting of the food types "measureless passion" and "transgressors".[13]

The 7 diet types

1. The health idealists:
Actively live out their ideals and beliefs. The center of life for these men and women is a conscious and creative life in harmony with nature. Their high standards are based on a very high quality of life, and health and fitness are very important to them. They buy fresh organic produce directly from producers and usually cook several times a day.

2. The problem conscious:
The traditional way of life of these men and women is characterized by a great health consciousness. Nevertheless, they suffer from diabetes, high cholesterol, high blood pressure and circulatory problems. They value quality and freshness, but insist on a reasonable price. They have a daily diet routine, are experienced and good cooks and prefer to eat at home.

3. The Nest warmer:

They are predominantly female and look for harmony in all areas of life. They find their center of their life in responsibility for the family. They are hedonists who live in balance with themselves and their environment. They value a fresh and balanced diet and are passionate cooks. For quality they are willing to pay a higher price.

4. The Harried:

They are always pressed for time and there is hardly any time in the day for them to eat. They are usually young to middle-aged men who have difficulty in securing a balance between work and leisure. They suffer from stress disorders such as insomnia, fatigue and obesity. Shopping for them is a chore and quality products play no role. Food is a secondary matter, and snacks and fast food are commonplace.

5. The modern multi-optionals:

They have high expectations of themselves and are also frequently under time pressure. They are constantly trying to create a good mix between me-time and we-time. They suffer from stress, so have the same symptoms as the harried. They eat irregularly, in a rush and often very late in the day. The modern multi-optionals want a wide range of fresh products and do not mind spending more for quality. Eating is a communal experience, but they can rarely enjoy it.

6. The transgressors:

They put more emphasis on quantity rather than quality and convenience over health. They are mostly younger, single men who are looking for fun and superficial enjoyment. Their health and fitness condition is poor and they often suffer from obesity. Shopping is perceived as a nuisance. They want food to be nearby and available at a cheap price. They consume their food unreflectively and partly in excessive portions. Microwave meals and frozen foods facilitate the preparation of their meals because they often lack cooking experience.

7. The passionless:
They are entirely dispassionate about many things in life. They are mostly men, who value material security and their own reputation. They have no health awareness and a good, balanced diet for them is not an issue. Shopping must be done as quickly as possible and be cheap. Simple meals, frozen meals and canned foods determine their diet. Cooking is related exclusively to nutrition and does not include any social aspect.

Except for the health idealists and the nest warmer, there is a clear gap, amongst Germans, between thought and action with regard to the health aspect in food issues. The moral values raised in public are only lived by a minority in everyday life.

These values include:

- the growing health orientation of consumers,
- an increasing focus on a work-life balance,
- the increasing pleasure orientation,
- the increasing need for variety, new impressions and experiences,
- raising awareness of environmental and animal welfare and sustainability and
- an ideal "back to nature" movement.[14]

Quality as a growing trend?

Only one in four consumers (26 percent) belongs to the group of "Quality Eater", which places a particularly high demand on the quality of food. In addition to good taste (89 percent) and high security (92 percent) this group wants food to be good for health (92 percent) and to cover sustainability issues such as animal welfare (81 percent).[15]

"Quality Eaters" are mostly female (62 percent) and older than 30 years, with a generally above average education and a higher household income. They often buy their groceries in farmers' markets and weekly markets. Freshness, naturalness, regionality, seasonality, Bio, transparency of origin and sustainability are all important to them. 67 percent of "Quality Eaters" belong to the health conscious group (Nest warmer, problem-conscious and health idealists), 28 percent are from the "short of time" group (harried and modern multi-optional), while five percent belong to the disinterested group (transgressor and passionless).

From diet to lifestyle

Things connected with one's diet are already an important element of one's lifestyle. No matter how big or expensive the kitchen, constantly there are new trends that make the kitchen a status symbol. Indeed, kitchen accessories are an important source of income for all furniture and furnishing stores. As such the food itself often becomes a minor matter. For example, the barbecue is a strong symbol of conviviality and hospitality. Grilling is considered the domain of men and the actual grill itself is considered a real status symbol. Most brands and equipment play a more important role than we realise.

The media make quite significant efforts to promote and support the trend to make nutrition a part of lifestyle. There is hardly a TV station that does not have a cooking show. Magazines with recipes have developed into glossy lifestyle magazines ranging from "Beef" for male meat eaters to "Vegan". Those magazines aimed at a vegan diet use this as a basis to promote a totally new lifestyle. It is thus not surprising that cookbooks regularly appear on bestseller lists and thereby turn cooks into media stars.

A special phenomenon is the sharp rise of food blogs on the Internet. The search engine Google has nearly 800 million records of amateurs and professionals presenting their recipes, their eating habits and lifestyles.

Those who see themselves as elite are already one step ahead. For them the term "food", with all its variations from slow food to Green food, is not as important as the new concept of "Healthy Wealth".

This describes a new health lifestyle, in which products are not the key status symbols, but the on-site spa. Avoiding and preventing diseases has a higher priority than their potential subsequent treatment. But one must be willing to pay more.[16]

Since all trends are passed down in society from top to bottom, we can therefore assume that this new health consciousness will soon be more widespread. In light of this, not only will people themselves benefit, but also service providers, consultants, and the food industry.

How the social environment shapes our eating habits

The pace of social change has accelerated in the past 30 years. Society is changing structurally, but also in everyday culture.

Among the facets of the profound structural changes that characterize nutritional behavior, are the following:

- the aging of society,
- the increase of single and two-person households,
- the growing proportion of working women,
- the development of prosperity in the various social classes,
- the increasing heterogeneity of the population.

At the same time changes in everyday culture include:

- the individualization of lifestyles,
- the partial dissolution of solid habits in daily organization, in leisure and consumer preferences
- the dissolution of fixed role patterns,
- the changed relationships between generations,
- the internationalization of experience among the population of the world,
- the mobility of the population,

- the abundance of options for information, leisure and consumption,
- the increase of time constraints.[17]

Destructuring the daily routine leads to the snack culture

One of the most important social factors influencing eating behavior is the gradual destructuring of daily routines. 35 percent of the total population and 41 percent of the working population continuously or frequently have an irregular daily routine. Among 20- to 29-year-olds, the percentage is as high as 52 percent. People with little regular daily routine rarely eat at set times of the day and not when they are hungry, but eat according to when they have windows of free time.[18]

So main meals are often replaced by snacks, especially among younger people. In Germany, more than two thirds of all under-30s eat something small now and then instead of a main meal. Others bridge the period between lunch and dinner with snacks. However, even these "Heavy Snackers" are increasingly interested in taste and health aspects.

As such, understanding of the definition of snack and snacking is increasingly lost. This is the conclusion the study "Snacking Motivations and Attitudes US 2015" by the market research firm Mintel.

For seven out of ten US adults, snacks include pizza or wraps and not just donuts. They regard all the food eaten in between meals as a snack. "Millennials" grab snacks much more often than older generations. A quarter of young adults in the United States eat four daily snacks in addition to their three main meals.[19]

Frequently, those with emotional problems and suffering from stress eat snacks. Most emotional eaters eat very quickly, in front of the refrigerator or in a standing position. They do not do it for the pleasure, but for the emotional comfort that the food gives them. For example, to briefly attenuate negative emotions such as fear and uncertainty a piece of chocolate is eaten. But such comfort eating is also followed by a guilty conscience.

Stress affects eating habits

A significant proportion of the population attests to a lack of discipline in diet. Almost one in five often eats something in between meals, without being hungry. One person in 10 eats a snack at least occasionally in response to frustration or stress.[20]

Researchers in Zurich have found that even mild stress reduces self-control. People who are under stress, have more problems controlling themselves than relaxed people. A person who starts the day under pressure and is comforted with this all day is more apt to eat unhealthily. In a laboratory test, some subjects were exposed to moderate stress by dipping their hand in ice water for three minutes. Afterwards all the subjects judged 180 different dishes, both for health and for taste. It was found that the people who had had the ice treatment were more likely to chose unhealthy food than the others. Clearly, this result was due to brain functions. It showed that stress affects the brain in several ways. In the first instance, signals are amplified, which push taste to the foreground, while other signals are attenuated, replacing the health aspect of food.[21]

Time pressure affects eating behavior

The destructuring of daily routines exacerbates a challenge particular to professionals: finding enough time every day for nutrition. For the most part, only dinner is given adequate time. 80 percent of all full-time professionals have lunch outside the home and, increasingly, breakfast. The "Mobile Eater" is the default result. Increasingly, these individuals replace breakfast with an on-the-go cup of coffee.[22] A study by Nestlé in 2009 determined that 56 percent of the working population partially succeed to eat as they actually wish and consider reasonable at the weekends.

Shortage of time also characterizes cooking habits. Nearly half of professionals try to save time in the week by not cooking and thus rely on convenience products. But shortage of time is only one of many reasons for convenience. Cooking with convenience foods is not only fast, but also easy and relatively cheap. Often no one in a household can now cook or wants to. Therefore one is limited to the heating up of a ready meal, whether on the stove, in the oven or in a microwave. This is especially the case in single and two-person households, the numbers of which are increasing.[23]

The other side of convenience is that it offers the opportunity to be varied in what one eats and to prepare sophisticated, multi-course meals with only moderate cooking skills. Convenience meals can also be individually refined thus fulfilling the desire of some households for self-realization.

The influence of diet on health

Today we stand on the threshold of a new era, in which the diet is no longer primarily considered as a power supply for the human body. It is a vital, active control instrument for people's own health and a long life. This knowledge will not only change food production profoundly, but also the behavior and habits at least of those people who want a long and healthy life for themselves and their children.

Science-based nutritional knowledge is still shockingly low even among the population of developed countries. This may be due, among other things, to the fact that nutrition research was long believed to have provided the necessary information for the prevention of diseases. But public health recommendations were accordingly flawed as they were based, as we have seen, often on error.

Using digital media, people can find easier access to more and more information around the world. The only problem is to distinguish correct and useful information from false facts presented in a scientific guise. Education today is far more than only being able to write, read and count. The ability of people to orient themselves in the electronic media without help, now has a disproportionately high importance.

Knowledge about nutrition has to be further developed and put on a scientific basis for all people, particulary children and adolescents. Today, there are still many shortcomings and misconceptions about the relationship between diet and health. But there is still also a lack of clear scientific evidence.

Gluten and lactose—The Free-from trend

Whereas a few years ago fat or vegetarian products were a symbol of healthy eating, this is now true of food that is lactose and gluten free. More and more people voluntarily refrain from lactose and gluten-containing products out of fear and because of the widespread nutritional half knowledge concerning their effect on health and improved well-being. The market for gluten-free products is growing rapidly, although they are on average 2.4 times as expensive as "normal products". In Germany, sales of gluten-free products are now amount to close to 60 million euros.[24] The official "Gluten Free Seal" of the German Celiac Society is today applied to many foods that have never even contained gluten.

In the US, this "Free-from-trend" is at an advanced stage. Almost one in three products claim they dispense with gluten. Many follow prominent actresses who report that a gluten-free diet has affected their wellbeing positively and they have thus lost weight. In fact, in healthy people, a gluten-free diet has no scientifically verifiable positive effects. The protein mixture of gluten is neither important nor harmful to the body. With a medical reason, avoiding gluten does not make anyone slimmer or healthier.

For patients who really have celiac disease, a form of gluten intolerance, a gluten-free diet, however, is vital. This autoimmune disease, according to estimates, affects no more than one percent of the population. In celiac patients, the consumption of gluten-containing foods leads to a defensive reaction from the immune system. The research is based on a genetic predisposition. However, all people with a genetic predisposition to celiac disease are far from being ill.

Very similar symptoms to celiac disease appear in people who have a gluten sensitivity. They often suffer from indigestion, but also migraines and depression, fatigue, and numbness and tingling in the limbs. The prevalence of gluten sensitivity varies from 1: 10,000 in Denmark and the United States and up to 1: 300 in Sweden and Great Britain.[25] People with gluten sensitivity can tolerate small amounts of gluten, while celiacs cannot.

The same trend for gluten-free products can be observed even with lactose-free foods. In South America, 50 percent of the population have lactose intolerance, while in North America (USA) it has been demonstrated in a study that 15 percent of white Americans, 53 percent of Mexican-Americans and 80 percent of African-Americans have lactose intolerance.[26]

Lactose is indeed an important nutrient. It is a double sugar, which must be split because the human body can only use its components of glucose and galactose. The digestive enzyme lactase splits the lactose in the small intestine. It is produced by the body. If this is not produced in sufficient quantities, it is called lactose intolerance.

People with lactose intolerance, who then ingest lactose, experience problems such as flatulence, abdominal pain or nausea. This is not a serious condition as with celiac disease, but rather a mood disorder. In evolutionary terms lactose intolerance was once the "normal state". From 7,500 years ago, people could not digest lactose and in many regions of Africa and Asia this is still the case. That Europeans and North Americans tolerate lactose is explained by a gene mutation. This means that their bodies produce large amounts of lactase and they can therefore drink milk without discomfort. The evolutionary advantage thus makes it possible to enjoy an additional source of food.[27]

Coffee is more than just a stimulant

Coffee is probably the most thoroughly researched food. Every year several hundred studies are published worldwide that deal with its effect on the human body. That there are repeatedly new findings, is also certainly due to the fact that more than 1,000 different substances have been identified in coffee, of which caffeine is the most famous. Alongside caffeine, coffee also contains carbohydrates, proteins, lipids and minerals.

Green coffee contains more than 80 different acids, while roasted and brewed coffee provides more than 800 different flavors in different combinations. Coffee is not just the result of using specific varieties and mixing them, but is also defined by the roasting process and the subsequent form of preparation.[28]

Caffeine is indeed the most widely consumed pharmacologically active substance, but it leads to hardly any dependence because it does not stimulate the reward system in the brain. Caffeine is present not only in the coffee but also in dark chocolate and tea. The effect of caffeine is felt about 20 minutes after drinking a cup of coffee. It acts against adenosine, a tiredness causing substance in the body. So caffeine suppresses fatigue and allows for faster response times. It also improves attention and memory, because it improves the storage of newly learned information.

Caffeine not only has positive effects on the brain, but also on the body. Research shows that it improves endurance. The risk of developing heart failure or heart attack or stroke is reduced. The same is true for cancers. As coffee contains many antioxidants alongside caffeine, coffee drinkers suffer less frequently from type 2 diabetes, Parkinson's disease and Alzheimer's disease.[29]

Anyone who believes that one cannot sleep well after drinking coffee is in most cases incorrect. What does not let a person sleep is the expectation associated with coffee. It may be, however, quite possible that coffee drinking in the evening shortens the length of sleep.[30]

The properties of spices

In 2015 two early studies published by the Nestlé Research Center (NRC) in collaboration with the Laboratory of Neuronal microcircuitry at the École Polytechnique Fédérale de Lausanne provided evidence that certain substances present in spices can have a positive effect on obesity, diabetes or epilepsy.[31] This finding now needs to be supported and deepened in further studies. Many traditional medical systems in the world have already experienced the positive effect of spices. However, corresponding documentary evidence is still lacking in studies.

The NRC has so far mainly examined cinnamon and peppermint. Scientists have also shown that certain drugs can dampen neural signals in the brain that may be associated with seizures: eugenol, for instance, is found in cloves, allspice leaves, but also in cinnamon or bay leaves, basil and nutmeg, similar to the capsaicin in Chilis or menthol in the peppermint plant. It is hoped that, with these agents, neurodegenerative diseases like Alzheimer's can be treated. The active ingredients in cinnamon also dampen the sensation of hunger. Research into the properties of spices is only in its early days.

From general nutrition advice to specific recommendations

Today the consumer can reliably be informed about which nutrients and what amounts the human body needs and what functions they perform. An example is the brochure "Healthy enjoyment. Food and drink for greater wellbeing" by Nestlé Germany.[32] But consumer and other non-profit organizations, as well as health insurance companies and government institutions, also offer a wealth of information from which the consumer can choose.

However, nutrition research still has limitations when it comes to metabolism, because it is very difficult to understand the entire processes and relationships regarding food that occur in the body. Genetic and epigenetic research has shown that the requirements that determine a healthy diet are not just age and daily physical activities. They also depend on the (epi) genetic makeup of a person. As we do not understand everything, general nutritional advice is only able to make basic statements and is not able to respond to the specific needs of individuals.

We now know that the diet of young women in the months before fertilization has a decisive role for the lifelong health of their child. The diet should be varied and balanced. It should contain sufficient amounts but not too much fat, sugar and salt micronutrients.

Most vitamins and all minerals can not be formed by the body itself, but are essential and must therefore be found in food. A lack of micronutrients can lead to numerous metabolic disorders that affect general growth, the structure of bones and teeth as well as the function of the immune system, the nerves and muscles. They play a role in the construction of hormones, enzymes and blood cells, and also affect the texture of the skin.[33]

Also, maternal malnutrition during pregnancy has an impact on the later development of the child. Maternal nutrition affects the epigenetic switch of the child, which controls the structure and functions of the body. Numerous studies have shown that being overweight as a mother and having a generally high weight gain during pregnancy significantly increases the risk of obesity of the child. The human fetus is particularly sensitive to a lack of nutrients, but also to excessive nutrient intake.

In children of mothers who had been starved during pregnancy, illnesses like diabetes, obesity or cardiovascular disease can develop more often than in other children. The fact that those effects themselves can be transferred to the grandchildren has been shown in a study on the impact of the "hunger winter" of 1944/45 in the Netherlands. The relationships between fasting during pregnancy and subsequent illnesses of children are currently being investigated further[34] in the context of two projects funded by the European Union.

The first 1,000 days are the most important

The first 1,000 days after conception are probably the most important in one's life. At this time, the course for the development of the immune system, the metabolic processes and brain development are provided. Instrumental in this is, as I have said elsewhere, a healthy microbiome.

The slogan "breast is best" summarizes concisely the results for all scientific research on the development of a child. Breast milk is rich in vital nutrients in the right amounts, and thus is the most suitable for the child. Studies have shown that breastfed babies are less overweight at school age. Weight gain in the later stages of life is predetermined in the first nine months of life.

Baby food served at the time of Henri Nestlé ensured the survival of an infant who could not tolerate breast milk. Today Nestlé is a leader in the development of infant formula for infants who can not be breastfed, to ensure a healthy start in life. The independent long-term study GINI has confirmed that infant food produced by Nestlé causes a reduction in the risk of allergy to milk protein.

The Nestlé Nutrition division offers high-quality, science-based nutritional products for mothers and babies. Correct feeding practices in early childhood are also impartant so that children get used to reasonable diet patterns.

Nestlé wants to empower people to make informed food choices. The company therefore supports mothers by providing extensive education and information materials. The interactive science education program "Start Healthy Stay Healthy" helps parents and carers to give good, developmentally appropriate nutrition in the crucial first 1,000 days of life of their child. It has been introduced in 25 countries, reaching, by the end of 2015, more than 20 million mothers and caregivers worldwide.

For medical professionals, the Nestlé Nutrition Institute (NNI) with its services and programs for nutrition education and nutrition-related health problems, is the largest source of nutritional information. By 2017, it intends to provide such information to twelve country-specific and several global websites in 10 languages and covering 50 countries.[35]

Proper nutrition for every age

In the subsequent lifetime of a child, it is not only an age appropriate diet that affects the eating behavior. In addition, food they grow up with can act as a role model for the education of a child. By the composition of their products and also through education and information, the food industry can help the parents.

This includes providing information on the product page about the reduction of sugar, salt and saturated fats and the importance of micronutrient fortification by using whole grains and fiber. 85 per cent of Nestlé breakfast cereals for children and adolescents include whole grains as the main ingredient.

For consumers, nutrition information is provided on the packaging and serving information on all products. In 2015 Nestlé used standard values for daily intake on 89.2 percent of all products and, to the extent legally permitted, 91.4 percent of children's products since daily recommended values on labels are not allowed by law in all countries.

It is necessary to point out the importance of a proper serving size for a healthy diet. It nonetheless remains difficult to change the consumption habits of consumers. Nestlé Portion Guidance is a voluntary initiative that connects international dietary guidelines and labeling requirements. At the end of 2015, 63.3% of all products contained serving information for children and families, and 76.9 percent of frequently consumed foods or snacks.

Vegetables are an important part of a healthy diet, but are not amongst the most favorite dishes of children. A study by the Nestlé Research Center has shown that children who helped their parents prepare the evening meal ate significantly more vegetables than those who did not. The involvement of children can therefore have a positive effect on the development of healthy eating habits.[36]

The Nestlé Healthy Kids Programme aims to encourage school-age children worldwide to adopt healthier eating and drinking habits and a healthier lifestyle. The transmission of knowledge about nutrition and health at the same time is promoted by competitions and workshops which stimulate physics activity amongst children. In 2015, this program was conducted in 84 countries together with nearly 285 partners, including national and local government organizations, NGOs and other institutions that deal with nutrition and health, as well as sports associations. By the end of 2015 more than eight million children were involved in the Healthy Kids programs.[37]

In early 2015 a completely new educational offering was launched by the Nestlé Museum Alimentaire, the Alimentarium Academy. This online platform provides tutorials and courses for children and their teachers or parents on food and nutrition, supplemented by games, videos and other activities. The teachers or parents have the opportunity to follow their children's progress and to participate in their training.[38]

But parents themselves must often first learn to eat properly. Contributing to this is the Maggi cooking class program that is currently running in 32 countries and pays special attention to cooking with whole grains and vegetables. An as yet largely unexplored area is the diet of adolescents and young adults.

How eating habits are formed

Eating habits are already formed in early childhood, so in the first few weeks and months they are learned and firmly anchored in the brain (hard-wired). This is not only perceived by the tongue on the basis of taste that characterizes and sustains later preferences, but also through complex information received from the mouth, throat and nasal passages. We also find that both the microbiome and genetic predispositions play an important role.

Of greater importance regarding our experience of taste than our other four senses of smell, sight, touch ("mouth feel") and hearing is the brain. Each of these senses sends messages to it which are then analyzed and interpreted. Only man has this brain-flavor system.[39] Food and drink target different areas of the brain according to the taste, smell and other sensory characteristics of the food. Scientists at the Nestlé Research Center use electroencephalography (EEG) to determine when and where in the brain the processing is done when the body and mind reacts to certain foods.

Even the appearance of food affects our perception: a feast for the eyes. A study by the Nestlé Research Center has revealed that taste better when volunteers have first been shown high-calorie foods, and that, conversely, taste seems worse after looking at low-calorie foods. The sight of caloric foods affects personal expectations of the taste before it is actually experienced.[40]

When today's adults over 30 years or older were babies, diet was mainly about ensuring nutrition and ensuring children were happy and satisfied. That these people today prefer sugary, salty and fatty foods should not be a surprise.

During childhood and as an adult, the sense of taste evolves. This is dependent on the regional food supply and also on the income situation and social status of families. With globalization the sense of taste has also changed. Thus, for example, Japanese food culture has spread strongly through Western countries, not least because more and more Japanese live there. In many parts of Europe, the socially better off acquired a taste for Japanese cuisine, which has been gradually "passed down" to those lower in the income scale. While there used to be only a few Japanese restaurants in the centers of cities, you can now buy Japanese food at discount stores throughout the provinces today. In the United States, Japanese cuisine came through California.

The development of taste establishes for each generation the basis of health and quality of life. But of course there is for all people at all times and at any age the opportunity to feel better, prevent disease or alleviate diseases through what we eat. But unhealthy eating habits have to change. This is extremely difficult.

Changing eating habits is difficult

To change the behavior of people is very difficult, and this is particularly true of their eating habits. Rational appeals to reason are only successful in a few people. The reason is that most decisions are made unconsciously and by simple heuristics, in which the rapid fulfillment of current need is paramount.

In connection with these heuristic decisions, simple patterns that are also perceptual distortions (cognitive biases), prevent behavioral changes. The majority of people prefer information that confirms their behavior rather than changes it. The present is more important than the future. Simple explanations are preferred to complex ones. All of this means that a lot of good scientific arguments go unheeded. How can one make a difference with adults?

The suggestion of behavioral economists is to give people little "nudges" in order to steer them in the right direction.[41] Such "nudges" are not requirements or prohibitions that restrict people's discretionary powers. They are simple, psychologically justified measures to convince more reasonable people, that they should also adopt healthier behavior. Especially in this regard, convenience plays a major role.

What has proven effective is making a salad bar in a cafeteria easier to find than the dessert display, or providing specifically subdivided shopping carts in supermarkets, in which half the space is allocated to healthy food. In fact, appropriate placement can commercially affect the habits and behaviors of consumers. But that alone is not enough. You have to offer consumers foods that are familiar to them and look, taste and are prepared exactly to suit their habits. And these foods must be made more healthy. This is the major challenge to the food industry.

CHAPTER 8:
MILESTONES ON THE WAY TO THE FUTURE

To live long and healthily, is the desire of all people. The fact that diet plays a crucial role has been made clear. For those who have a lower income, this means providing sufficient healthy food enriched with micronutrients and clean water. For those with a higher income, the outlook is quite different. Progress in the life sciences and the strategic reorientation of the food industry opens up countless new opportunities for a longer, better life. It is moreover important to find solutions to challenges created by the negative effects of past successes: Too much available food and perverse incentives and beliefs led by the middle of the 1990s to many people overeating, which has been strongly associated with the massive increase in metabolic health related diseases such as diabetes, obesity and cardiovascular.

Industrially produced food in the context of customized diets for specific populations can provide clear health benefits over simple and seemingly "natural" foods. However, the cost and value per calorie consumed of such foods will rise. What will make these foods more expensive is the amount of scientific research that will go into their development, and the differentiation and the complex manufacturing processes used to obtain the flavor and the taste experience.

To meet the needs of the growing world population in the future also requires a more conscious use of natural resources, particularly water and arable land. Incentives must be created to use less water, ensure less clearance of forests for farmland and to restrict polluting the environment. Any reduction in the use of resources must be rewarded unlike the unbridled exploitation of nature. We know that this is possible today. For example, millions will be helped by small farmers increasing their yields from agriculture and livestock, without using more resources.

In improving the diet of people there are many obstacles that have to be overcome, many of which are anchored in the mind. The industrial science-based manufacture of food will not just result in the future worldwide availability of food. How we eat, depends on the relevant cultural, religious and social conditions in which we live. Add to this the natural environmental conditions that determine our way of life, and the personal genetic features that distinguish people from each other.

Especially in the field of nutrition, there are perceptual distortions in the populations of developed countries, which are partly ideological and partly justified by contradictory scientific findings. For example, the idea that raw food is less healthy has turned out to be largely wrong.

Beliefs can change perceptions and even affect metabolic processes. That is why it is so important to provide new scientific evidence on a broad basis. Only through a new holistic approach to thinking and a new quality in terms of a long and healthy life are we able to reach our goals. How the right diet will look like in the future can be seen already though it is still in its infancy. It remains for industry and society to formulate new standards of quality, both in the areas of the use of natural resources as well as personalized diet and its implementation.

What is conceivable, what is possible?

Both the current and future food research on the molecular basis has to work with very precise and detailed questions to get accurate answers, which can then be generalized again. The Life Sciences have now proved that the "optimal diet" of people varies considerably.[1]

Nutrigenomics and Nutri(epi)genetics will contribute to the scientific basis for personal, optimal nutrition. The sequencing and methylation techniques are becoming more widespread and easily accessible. Although people can get valuable information from their personal (epi)genetic code already, the implementation and application of the wealth of new information will still take a long time to complete.

Food with new quality

The revolution in food production in the coming decades will not primarily be based on the fact that we will use algae as a basis for new plant foods or that we might gain certain proteins from insects, nor that we will produce in vitro meat. All of these topics are about the replacement of existing raw materials by others with similar characteristics and of similar quality, sometimes with the aim of protecting resources. The more profound revolution is that we are giving food a completely new quality from the point of health. New foods will be directed against the major diseases: Alzheimer's, depression, diabetes, cardiovascular problems and obesity.[2]

The future will not be in "superfoods", such as the chia seeds, which the Maya and Aztecs used. Such superfood is nothing more than short-term fads for short-term profit. Maybe superfood for consumers can have some placebo effects, but this then evaporates when a new consumer trend appears.[3]

Many start-ups in the US are trying to reinvent food by developing environmentally compatible plant-based "art food". At the forefront of this movement are companies like Beyond Meat and Hampton Creek. Beyond Meat provides art food derived from pea proteins and Hampton Creek produces mayonnaise and cookies from vegetable substitutes. Both companies have gained influential investors.[4]

Another route has been suggested by the electrical engineer Robert Rhinehart. With his development of the art food called Soylent composed of the English words "Soy" and "Lentils" he is looking to save time and money for himself and his colleagues from the computer industry. Why waste a lot of time shopping and cooking, or going to a restaurant when it is possible at work and everywhere else to take a liquid food with you for the price of four dollars a meal, that provides the body with all that it needs? One need never have to worry about food again and can concentrate on all the things that, in his view, are really important.[5]

Soylent is a brownish powder, which is mixed with water. It tastes bland and has a slimy "mouthfeel". How large the number of consumers is who want to eat in this way, has yet to be seen.

The benefits of genetic testing are not yet clear

It is very likely that more and more people will have their genome decoded so as to know their personal health risks and how to prevent them. Genome sequencing is already available at a cost of around 1,000 dollars but this is likely to fall in a few years, even perhaps to as low as ten dollars.[6]

The benefits associated with this are, however, not yet fully known. It is, after all, not just about the decoding of the personal genome, but also the genome of the much more complex microbiome, and, furthermore, appropriate digital devices and their interlinkage are needed to make completely new health recommendations.

With small "Wearables", i.e. portable Internet-enabled devices, such as a health watch, a sphygmomanometer or an ear thermometer, different bodies of data (e.g., blood pressure, pulse, blood sugar, body temperature, rest, exercise and sleep phases) can be collected and sent via Bluetooth to a smartphone app. This will monitor our health data and recommend resulting nutrition and practices.[7]

This may lead to a significant change in lifestyle for large sections of the population. People over 40 will, in particular, be increasingly interested in fitness bracelets, to analyze heart problems, high blood pressure or, invasively, blood glucose levels. This will also enable GPs to access information that is not available to them today.

Big Data opens new possibilities

Knowing more about our bodies and our food presents a new framework of self-determination. Lifelogging devices will record the entire daily routine of their users, from sleeping to waking up so as to compare with previous stages. Then there is the need, however, to implement the resulting nutritional recommendations correctly.[8]

The "Internet of Things" increasingly provides opportunities to exchange data through a variety of technical devices. It offers companies the opportunity to develop new products or systems which can personalize food more than ever without the costs becoming excessive. The real challenge is to use this data to detect through a portable sensor, how many calories are consumed during the day, and then plan the next meal so that these calories and nutrients are taken into account and limits set. The opportunities of the digital revolution will continue to increase in the coming years.

Thus the Nestlé project, which was named "Iron Man" by the press, intends to revolutionize diets. Using a capsule similar to a Nespresso, people will be able to take individual nutrient cocktails or prepare their food via 3D printers according to electronically recorded health recommendations. That sounds more like science fiction too, but it could be a reality within the next ten years. Personalized working kitchen utensils, personalized shopping recommendations, commercial and personalized menu recommendations in restaurants, schools and workplaces, will no longer be a utopia.

APPENDIX

WHO—guideline and values for the consumption of sugar, salt and trans fats

The guidelines of the World Health Organisation contain fundamental statements about a healthy diet and special guidelines for the consumption of sugar, salt and fats for children and adults. Sugar is understood as referring to so-called "free sugars", that are mixed with food and drink, and not to the natural sugar content of fruit, vegetables and milk, which is not regarded by WHO as harmful. On the subject of salt, this includes the consumption of potassium (potassium) and sodium (sodium).

These excerpts are reproduced from the original texts.

1.   Healthy diet

A healthy diet for adults contains:

- Fruits, vegetables, legumes (e.g. lentils, beans), nuts and whole grains (e.g. unprocessed maize, millet, oats, wheat, brown rice).
- At least 400 g (5 portions) of fruits and vegetables a day. Potatoes, sweet potatoes, cassava and other starchy roots are not classified as fruits or vegetables.

- Less than 10% of total energy intake from free sugars which is equivalent to 50 g (or around 12 level teaspoons) for a person of healthy body weight consuming approximately 2000 calories per day, but ideally less than 5% of total energy intake for additional health benefits. Most free sugars are added to foods or drinks by the manufacturer, cook or consumer, and can also be found in sugars naturally present in honey, syrups, fruit juices and fruit juice concentrates.
- Less than 30% of total energy intake from fats. Unsaturated fats (e.g. found in fish, avocado, nuts, sunflower, canola and olive oils) are preferable to saturated fats (e.g. found in fatty meat, butter, palm and coconut oil, cream, cheese, ghee and lard. Industrial trans fats (found in processed food, fast food, snack food, fried food, frozen pizza, pies, cookies, margarines and spreads) are not part of a healthy diet.
- Less than 5 g of salt (equivalent to approximately 1 teaspoon) per day and use iodized salt.

WHO fact sheet N°394; updated September 2015
http://www.who.int/mediacentre/factsheets/fs394/en/

2. Information note about intake of sugars recommended in the WHO guideline for adults and children

The World Health Organization's new Guideline: Sugars intake for adults and children recommends reduced intake of free sugars throughout the life course. In both adults and children, the intake of free sugars should be reduced to less than 10% of total energy intake. A further reduction to below 5% of total energy intake would provide additional health benefits.

Free sugars versus intrinsic sugars

Recommendations in the guideline focus on documented health effects associated with the intake of "free sugars". These include monosaccharides and disaccharides added to foods by the manufacturer, cook or consumer, and sugars naturally present in honey, syrups, fruit juices and fruit juice concentrates.

Free sugars are different from intrinsic sugars found in whole fresh fruits and vegetables. As no reported evidence links the consumption of intrinsic sugars to adverse health effects, recommendations in the guideline do not apply to the consumption of intrinsic sugars present in whole fresh fruits and vegetables.

Strong recommendations

The recommendations to reduce the intake of free sugars and to do so throughout the life course are based on analysis of the latest scientific evidence. This evidence shows, first, that adults who consume less sugars have lower body weight and, second, that increasing the amount of sugars in the diet is associated with a comparable weight increase. In addition, research shows that children with the highest intakes of sugar-sweetened drinks are more likely to be overweight or obese than children with a low intake of sugar-sweetened drinks.

The recommendation is further supported by evidence showing higher rates of dental caries when the intake of free sugars is above 10% of total energy intake compared with an intake of free sugars below 10% of total energy intake.

Based on the quality of supporting evidence, these recommendations are ranked by WHO as "strong": they can be adopted as policy in most situations. Countries can act on these recommendations by developing food-based dietary guidelines, taking into consideration locally available food and dietary customs.

Other policy options include food and nutrition labelling, consumer education, regulation of marketing of food and non-alcoholic beverages that are high in free sugars, and fiscal policies targeting foods that are high in free sugars. Individuals can implement these recommendations by changes in their food choices.

Further reduction: a conditional recommendation

Given the nature of existing studies, the recommendation of reducing intake of free sugars to below 5% of total energy is presented as "conditional" in the WHO system for issuing evidence-based guidance.

Few epidemiological studies have been undertaken in populations with a low sugars intake. Only three national population-wide studies allow a comparison of dental caries with sugars intakes of less than 5% of total energy intake versus sugars intakes of more than 5% of total energy intake, but less than 10% of total energy intake.

These population-based ecological studies were conducted during a period when sugars availability dropped dramatically from 15 kg per person per year before the Second World War to a low of 0.2 kg per person per year in 1946. This "natural experiment", which demonstrated a reduction in dental caries, provides the basis for the recommendation that reducing the intake of free sugars below 5% of total energy intake would provide additional health benefits in the form of reduced dental caries.

The treatment of dental diseases absorbs from 5% to 10% of health budgets in wealthy countries. Dental caries goes largely untreated in lower income countries, where the cost would exceed all financial resources available for the health care of children.

WHO issues conditional recommendations even when the quality of evidence may not be strong on the issues related to public health importance. A conditional recommendation is one where the desirable effects of adhering to the recommendation probably outweigh the undesirable effects but these tradeoffs could not be clarified; therefore, stakeholder dialogue and consultations are needed before the recommendation is implemented as policy.

http://www.who.int/nutrition/publications/guidelines/
sugar_intake_information_note_en.pdf

WHO guidance on dietary salt and potassium

Adults should consume less than 2,000 mg of sodium, or 5 grams of salt, and at least 3,510 mg of potassium per day, according to new guidelines issued by the WHO. A person with either elevated sodium levels and low potassium levels could be at risk of raised blood pressure which increases the risk of heart disease and stroke.

Sodium is found naturally in a variety of foods, including milk and cream (approximately 50 mg of sodium per 100 g) and eggs (approximately 80 mg/100 g). It is also found, in much higher amounts, in processed foods, such as bread (approximately 250 mg/100 g), processed meats like bacon (approximately 1,500 mg/100 g), snack foods such as pretzels, cheese puffs and popcorn (approximately 1,500 mg/100 g), as well as in condiments such as soy sauce (approximately 7,000 mg/100 g), and bouillon or stock cubes (approximately 20,000 mg/100 g).

Potassium-rich foods include: beans and peas (approximately 1,300 mg of potassium per 100 g), nuts (approximately 600 mg/100 g), vegetables such as spinach, cabbage and parsley (approximately 550 mg/100 g) and fruits such as bananas, papayas and dates (approximately 300 mg/100 g). Processing reduces the amount of potassium in many food products. Currently, most people consume too much sodium and not enough potassium.

"Elevated blood pressure is a major risk for heart disease and stroke—the number one cause of death and disability globally," says Dr Francesco Branca, Director of WHO's Department of Nutrition for Health and Development. "These guidelines also make recommendations for children over the age of 2. This is critical because children with elevated blood pressure often become adults with elevated blood pressure."

The guidelines are an important tool for public health experts and policymakers as they work in their specific country situations to address non-communicable diseases such as heart disease, stroke, diabetes, cancer and chronic respiratory diseases. Public health measures to reduce sodium and increase potassium consumption and thereby decrease the population's risk of high blood pressure and heart disease can include food and product labelling, consumer education, updating national dietary guidelines, and negotiating with food manufacturers to reduce the amount of salt in processed foods.

http://www.who.int/mediacentre/news/notes/2013/salt_potas sium_20130131/en/

Total fat and fatty acids

Interim Summary of Conclusions and Dietary Recommendations on Total Fat & Fatty Acids; from the Joint FAO/WHO Expert Consultation on Fats and Fatty Acids in Human Nutrition, 10–14 November, 2008, WHO, Geneva

There are the inherent limitations with the convention of grouping fatty acids based only on the number of double bonds, i.e. saturated fatty acids (SFA), monounsaturated fatty acids (MUFA) and polyunsaturated fatty acids (PUFA) insofar as describing the effects of fatty acids on human health and in developing dietary recommendations. The large body of epidemiological evidence about total fats, fatty acids, and human health apply these groupings and show that the major groups of fatty acids are associated with different health effects. However, the consultation experts recognise that individual fatty acids within each broad classification of fatty acids may have unique biological properties and health effects. This has relevance in making global recommendations because intakes of the individual fatty acids that make up the broad groupings will differ across regions of the world depending on the predominant food sources of total fats and oils. The experts also recognized that in spite of these limitations, the scientific community in general and an increasing proportion of the general population continue to use the groupings based on chemical structure and thus, there would be disadvantages in abandoning them. Moreover, few countries have food composition databases that enable dietary assessment of individual fatty acid intake.

Summary of Total Fat and Fatty Acid Requirements for Adults, Infants (0–24 months) and Children (2–18 years)

There was convincing evidence that energy balance is critical to maintaining healthy body weight and ensuring optimal nutrient intakes, regardless of macronutrient distribution expressed in energy percentage (%E). The requirements on total fat and different fatty acid groups are summarized in the tables below: the first for adults and the second for infants and children. It is emphasized that requirements should be tailored to individuals and that the general requirements for certain groups, e.g. children and elderly subjects, have not yet been adequately established.

Minimum total fat intakes for adults:

- 15%E to ensure adequate consumption of total energy, essential fatty acids, and fat soluble vitamins for most individuals.
- 20%E for women of reproductive age and adults with BMI < 18.5, especially in developing countries in which dietary fat may be important to achieve adequate energy intake in malnourished populations.
- Maximum total fat intakes for adults:
- 30–35%E for most individuals

Conclusions and Recommended dietary requirements for trans-fatty acid intake (TFA)

The Consultation devoted substantial time and discussion to the issue of trans-fatty acid (TFA) but in doing so drew heavily from the conclusions of the recently concluded and published reports of the WHO Scientific Update on trans fatty acids (Nishida & Uauy, EJCN, Vol 63, Suppl 2, 2009). There is convincing evidence that TFA from commercial partially hydrogenated vegetable oils (PHVO) increase CHD risk factors and CHD events—more so than had been thought in the past. There also is probable evidence of an increased risk of fatal CHD and sudden cardiac death in addition to an increased risk of metabolic syndrome components and diabetes. In promoting the removal of TFA, which are predominantly a by-product of industrial processing (partial hydrogenation) usually in the form of PHVO, particular attention must be given to what would be their replacement; this is a challenge for the food industry. It was noted that among adults, the estimated average daily ruminant TFA intake in most societies is low. The experts acknowledged the current recommendation of a mean population intake of TFA of less than 1%E may need to be revised in light of the fact that it does not fully take into account the distribution of intakes and thus the need to protect substantial subgroups from having dangerously high intakes. This could well lead to the need to remove partially hydrogenated fats and oils from the human food supply.

http://www.who.int/nutrition/topics/FFA_human_nutrition/en/

NOTES

Introduction

1 http://ourworldindata.org/data/population-growth-vital-statistics/life-expectancy/and http://www.geoba.se/population.php?pc=world&type =15
2 cf. Maddison, Angus: The World Economy—A Millenial Perspective, Paris 2001
3 http://www.who.int/gho/mortality_burden_disease/life_tables/situation_trends/en/
4 Nestlé CT-ENT Charts Economics and Context ob/tv #4

Chapter 1:
On the way to feeding the future

1 cf. Naisbitt, John: Megatrends. 10 Perspektiven, die unser Leben verändern werden, Munich 1985
2 http://de.statista.com/statistik/daten/studie/2995/umfrage/entwick lung-der-weltweiten-mobilfunkteilnehmer-seit-1993
3 cf. United Nations Department of Economic and Social Affairs Popular Division: World Population Prospects. The 2015 Revision. Key findings and Advance Tables, New York 2015
4 cf. Transgenerational Design Matters, The Demographics of Aging, http://transgenerational.org/demographics.html
5 cf. http://www.un.org/depts/german/milleniumMDG%20Report%20 2013_german.pdf
6 cf. ibid.
7 cf. ibid

8   http://www.census.gov/population/projections/data/national/2012/
    summarytables.html
9   cf. Zukunftsinstitut https://www.zukunftsinstitut.de
10 cf. ibid.
11 cf. ibid.
12 cf. ibid.
13 cf. World Health Summit http://www.worldhealthsummit.org/World
    Health Summit
14 U.S. Department of Health & Human Services http://www.cdc.gov/
    chronicdisease/
15 cf. International Diabetes Federation (IDF): IDF Diabetes Atlas 2014
16 cf. UN World Population Prospects
17 cf. http://www.spiegel.de/gesundheit/diagnose/demenz-zahl-der-erkran
    kten-steigt-in-zukunft-rasant-a-937318.html
18 cf. stern.de, 10.10.2010
19 cf. WHO Global status report of noncommunicable diseases 2014
20 cf. pharmazeutische-zeitung.de Ausgabe 18, 2011
21 cf. Zeit Magazin 11/2013
22 cf. Briesen, Detlef: Das gesunde Leben. Ernährung und Gesundheit seit
    dem 18. Jahrhundert. Frankfurt/New York 2010, S. 233ff
23 cf. Tomorrow Focus Media, http://www.forward-adgroup.de/fileadmin/
    customer_files/public_files/downloads/studien/TFM_SocialTrends_
    Gesundheit.pdf?PHPSESSID=295e1c582953f740d0d9fc8d12bda56c
24 cf. healthon.de
25 cf. Nestlé Zukunftsforum/tns infratest: NZF-Factbook II, Consumer
    Confusion
26 cf. UN/ESA http://esa.un.org/unup
27 Leitzmann, Claus/Cannon, Geoffrey: Die Gießener Erklärung zum Pro-
    jekt "Die neue Ernährungswissenschaft", in: Ernährungs-Umschau 53
    (2006) Heft 2
28 cf. ibid.
29 cf. Briesen
30 cf. ibid
31 cf. Bundesministerium für Bildung und Forschung: Stoffwechselfor-
    schung. Wie Ernährung und Gene auf die Gesundheit wirken. Bonn,
    Berlin 2008
32 cf. ibid
33 cf. Constantin, Nathalie/Wahli, Walter: Die Nutrigenomik oder der Kö-
    nigsweg zu einer präventiven Ernährung, in SVDE (Schweizerischer
    Verband diplomierter Ernährungsberater/innen) ASDD Info 6/2013
34 cf. Ahmed, Farooq, Tales of adversity, in: Nature, Vol. 468, 23/30 Decem-
    ber 2010

35 cf. EpiGen Global Research Consortium, Press Release 4th February
2015 http://www.epigengrc.com/news

Chapter 2:
From the beginnings of industrial food production to today

1 cf. Teuteberg, Hans J./Wiegelmann, Günter: Nahrungsgewohnheiten in
der Industrialisierung des 19. Jahrhunderts, Berlin 2005
2 cf. ibid.
3 cf. ibid.
4 sen, p. 15
5 cf. http://www.vulkane.net/vulkanismus/katastrophen/tambora.html
6 cf. http://www.welt.de/kultur/history/article106227344/Es-war-ein-Pilz-
der-eine-Million-Iren-toetete.html
7 cf. http://suite101.de/article/steckruebenwinter-im-ersten-weltkrieg-a62
563
8 http://www.zeit.de/2012/17/Riesenreich-China/seite-4
9 Briesen, p. 37
10 United Nations (UN), 1973, The Determinants and Consequences of Population Trends, p.10.
11 Briesen, p. 37
12 Briesen, p. 38
13 cf. Briesen, pp. 58ff
14 cf. Technoseum Landesmuseum für Technik und Arbeit in Mannheim
(Hrsg): Unser täglich Brot ... Die Industrialisierung der Ernährung, :
Katalog zur Ausstellung vom 28.10.2011—29.4.2012, Mannheim, 2011.
15 cf. Briesen, p. 58
16 cf. Nestlé AG (Hrsg.): Heer, Jean: Nestlé hundertfünfundzwanzig Jahre
von 1866 bis 1991, Vevey 1991
17 cf. Technoseum
18 cf. ibid.
19 cf. ibid.
20 cf. Briesen, p. 59
21 cf. http://www.nestle-marktplatz.de/view/Marken/Libbys
22 cf. http://www.campbellsoupcompany.com/about-campbell/
23 cf. http://www.heinzketchup.de/UeberHeinz/OurHistory
24 cf. http://www.weck.de/index.php/ueber-uns

25 cf. Briesen, p. 62

26 cf. Brisen, p. 47

27 cf. Brisen, p. 65

28 cf. IDF Faktenblatt des Internationalen Milchwirtschaftsverbandes (IDF) Februar 2013

29 cf. http://www.famoustexans.com/GailBorden.htm

30 Notizen von Brian Suter, Generaldirektor Forschung und Entwicklung Nestlé AG 1987–1997, and *Nestlé hundertfünfundzwanzig Jahre*

31 cf. http://www.britannica.com/biography/Hippolyte-Mege-Mouries

32 cf. http://www.unilever.de/ueberuns/unseregeschichte/

33 cf. Technoseum

34 cf. Briesen, p. 63

35 cf. König, p. 158

36 cf. König, p. 137 and p. 158

37 cf. Technoseum

38 cf. http://cailler.ch/de/alles-uber-cailler/geschichte/19-jahrhundert/

39 cf. http://cailler.ch/de/alles-uber-cailler/geschichte/20-jahrhundert/

40 cf. König, p. 143

41 cf. http://www.the-linde-group.com/internet.global.thelindegroup.glo bal/de/images/chronik_d%5B1%5D16_9855.pdf

42 cf. Technpseum

43 cf. http://www.biography.com/people/clarence-birdseye-9213147

44 cf. König, p. 145

45 cf. König, p. 138

46 cf. König, p. 172

47 cf. Briesen, p. 60

48 cf. König, p. 174

49 cf. Spiekermann, p. 362

50 cf. http://de.mintel.com/pressestelle/china-ueberholt-usa-als-weltweit-groesster-eiscreme-markt

51 cf. http://euroglaces.eu/en/Facts-figures/General Overview/

52 cf. Pendergrast, Mark: Für Gott und Coca-Cola. Die unautorisierte Geschichte der Coca-Cola Company. München 1993

53 cf. Heimann, Jim: Car Hops and Curb service. A History of American Drive-In Restaurants 1920–1960. Chronicle Books/Edition Stemmle, Kilchberg 1996.

54 cf. König, p. 178

55 tps://www.aid.de/verbraucher/convenience.php

56 cf. Technoseum, p. 257

57 cf. Fenner Thomas: Flagschiff Nescafé – Nestlés Aufstieg zum größten Lebensmittelkonzern der Welt, Baden 2015

58 cf. http://www.kelloggs.de/de_DE/who-we-are-landing/our-history.html

59 cf. Brisen, p. 63

60 cf. Porter, Michael u.a.: Nestlé`s Creating Shared Value Strategy, Harvard Business School N9–716–4229

61 cf. Nestlé hundertfünfundzwanzig Jahre und Nestlé (Hrsg.): Pfiffner, Albert/Renk, Hans-Jörg: Wandel als Herausforderung. Nestlé 1990–2005, Cham und Vevey 2007

62 cf. Nestlé: Nestlé in society—Creating Shared Value and meeting our commitments, 2014

Chapter 3:
How can a growing world population stay healthy and live longer?

1 cf. Briesen

2 cf. UN World Population Prospects 2015

3 http://esa.un.org/unpd/wup/highlights/wup2014-highlights.pdf

4 cf. Lang/Heasman, p. 18ff

5 cf. Nestlé in der Gesellschaft. Gemeinsame Wertschöpfung und umsere sozialen Verpflichtungen 2015

6 cf. Fraunhofer-Institut

7 cf. Fraunhofer-Institut

8 cf. ibid.

9 cf. ibid.

10 cf. FoodDrinkEurope

11 cf. USDA Research Investments

12 cf. https://www.landwirtschaft-bw.info/pb/MLR.Ernaehrung,Lde/Startseite/Empfehlungen/Kohlenhydrate_+Fett+und+Eiweiss+_+Hauptnaehrstoffe+im+Ueberblick/?LISTPAGE=1063164

13 cf. Nestlé: Nestlé Policy on Micronutrient Fortification of Foods & Beverages

14 cf. Nestlé in der Gesellschaft. Gemeinsame Wertschöpfung und unsere sozialen Verpflichtungen 2015

15 cf. Nestlé: Nutrition landscaping for effective fortification http://www.nestle.com/Media/NewsAndFeatures/

16 quoted from Biesalski, Taschenatlas Ernährung

17 cf. Leitzmann, Ernährung in Prävention

18 cf. ibid.

19 cf. http://www.fh-erfurt.de/lgf/fileadmin/GB/Dokumente/Forschung/Bioaktive_Substanzen_im_Gemuese.pdf

20 cf. ibid.

21 cf. Nestlé in der Gesellschaft. Gemeinsame Wertschöpfung und unsere sozialen Verpflichtungen 2015

22 Conversation with Stephan Palzer, Vice President Global Research & Development Manager Beverage Strategic Business Unit

23 Conversation with Thomas Beck, Director of Nestlé Research Center

24 Conversation with Stephan Palzer

25 cf. FoodDrinkEurope

26 cf. ibid.

27 cf. ibid.

28 cf. United States Department of Agriculture Economic Research Service

29 cf. ibid.

30 cf. ibid.

31 cf. Confederation of the food and drink industries of the EU CIAA

32 cf. FoodDrinkEurope

33 cf. FoodDrinkEurope

34 cf. ibid.

35 Nestlé Jahresbericht 2014

36 http://www.spektrum.de/lexikon/geographie/agrobusiness/191

37 cf. Nestlé, Wandel als Herausforderung, p. 58ff

38 cf. Metro-Handelslexikon

39 cf. Nestlé, Wandel als Herausforderung, p. 74

40 cf. ibid.

41 Cf. European Commission, Food Safety

42 http://www.who.int/mediacentre/factsheets/fs330/en/

43 World Health Organization http://www.who.int/bulletin/volumes/93/4/15-154831/en/

44 European Food Information Council (EUFIC) und WHO Codex Alimentarus Commission http://www.who.int/mediacentre/events/meetings/2015/codex-alimentarius-commission/en/ und http://www.who.int/mediacentre/factsheets/fs399/en/

45 cf. PWC Deutschland

Chapter 4:
Life Sciences and the revolution of biology, nutrition and health

1 cf. http://www.planet-wissen.de/natur/forschung/epigenetik/pwwbepigenetik100.html

2   Conversation with Emmanuel E. Baetge, Direktor des Nestlé Institute of Health Sciences

3   cf. Kussmann/Dean et al.: http://www.research.nestle.com/resources/downloads/Documents/Nestle%C3%A9%20White%20paper%20Nutrigenomics %20FINAL.pdf

4   cf. Kussmann & Van Bladeren 2011

5   cf. Kussmann & Fay 2008

6   cf. Kussmann, Krause et al. http://onlinelibrary.wiley.com/doi/10.1111/j.1753–4887.2010.00326.x/abstract

7   cf. http://www.research.nestle.com/newscenter/news/nestl%C3%A9researchcenterannouncescollaborationwithepigen,aleadingconsortium-forepigeneticsresearch

8   http://www.nestle.com/media/newsandfeatures/nestle-research-epigenetics

9   cf. http://earlybirddiabetes.org./findings.php

10 cf. Kussmann/Dean et al.: http://www.research.nestle.com/resources/downloads/Documents/Nestle%C3%A9%20White%20paper%20Nutrigenomics %20FINAL.pdf

11 cf. Nestlé, Unlocking the metabolic 'master switch' http://www.nestle.com/media/newsandfeatures/ampk-metabolic-master-switch

12 http://www.vfa-bio.de/vb-de/aktuelle-themen/forschung/mikrobiom.html

13 cf. Charisius/Friebe, 2014

14 cf. Kahlert/Müller, 2014

15 cf. Kussmann/Van Bladeren, 2011

16 cf. ibid.

17 cf. http://www.diaetologen.at/fileadmin/user_upload/documents/Kongress/Abstracts_Ernaehrungskongress/Holzer.pdf

18 cf. Focus Nr. 30/2013, Wo die Gesundheit sitzt, p. 79 ff.

19 cf. Der Spiegel Wissen 4/2013, Bauchsache pp. 108 ff

20 Antony Fodor, zitiert in www.spiegel.de vom 14.08.2012

21 cf. Charisius/Friebe, 2014

22 cf. ibid.

23 cf. Kussmann & Van Bladeren 2011

24 cf. ibid., p. 112

25 Nestlé Nutrition Institute https://www.nestlenutrition-institute.org/country/in/News/Pages/the-pattern-of-infants-gut-bacteria-biomarkers-of-future-food-allergy.aspx)

26 cf. Agency for Science, Technology and Research http://www.a-star.edu.sg/Media/News/Press-Releases/ID/3816/Infant-gut-microbiota-linked-with-gestation-duration-delivery-method-and-healthy-weight-gain.aspx

27 cf. NIHS News from the Institute NIHS 3.5.2015 https://www.nestleins titutehealthsciences.com/news/newsinstitute/nestl%C3%A9%20institu te%20of%20health%20sciences%20steps%20up%20a%20gear%20 in%20the%20fight%20against%20muscle%20loss%20in%20old%20 age

28 cf. https://www.nestlehealthscience.com/ newsroom/press-releases/the- role-of-nutrition-in-dementia-prevention-and-management

29 cf. Verbraucherzentrale Bundesverband e.V. (vzbv)(Hrsg.): Essen im Al- ter, 2004.

30 cf. https://www.nestleinstitutehealthsciences.com/news/newsinstitute/ press-release-three

Chapter 5:
The responsibility of the food industry

1 Conversation with Stefan Catsicas, Executive Vice President Nestlé S.A., Chief Technology Officer, Head of Innovation, Technology, Research and Development

2 http://www.euromonitor.com/passport

3 cf. Fraunhofer-Institut

4 cf. Frankfurter Allgemeine Zeitung, 25. October 2014, Die Welt ist dem Silicon Valley nicht genug

5 cf. https://www.futuremanagementgroup.com/.../Transhumanismus?

6 cf. https://www.nestlehealthscience.de/Ern%C3%A4hrungsthemen/ HCP/Kau-und-Schluckst%C3%B6rung

7 cf. http://www.nestle.de/themenwelten/news-storys/ernaehrung-der- zukunft-stoffwechsel

8 cf. GEO kompakt Nr. 42, 2015, p.30

9 http://www.nestle.de/themenwelten/news-storys/lebensmittel-solar- impulse

Chapter 7:
The responsibility of each individual

1 cf. Alcock et al.: Bioessays 36: 940–949, www.bioessays.de

2   cf. ibid.

3   cf. ibid.

4   cf. ibid.

5   cf. ibid.

6   cf. ibid.

7   Conversation with Thomas Beck.

8   cf. Nestlé Deutschland AG, Studie 2012

9   cf. www.heart.org und Teicholz

10 cf. Belasco

11 cf. Nestlé Deutschland AG, Studie 2009

12 cf. ibid.

13 cf. Nestlé Deutschland AG, Studie 2012

14 cf. Nestlé Deutschland AG, Studie 2009

15 cf. Nestlé Deutschland AG, Studie 2012

16 Bain Company, Pressemitteilung, 30. January 2014

17 cf. Nestlé Deutschland AG, Studie 2009

18 cf. Nestlé Deutschland AG, Studie 2011

19 cf. Mintel http://mintel.com

20 cf. Nestlé Deutschland AG, Studie 2009

21 cf. http://www.welt.de/gesundheit/psychologie/article144879242/
    Schon-leichter-Stress-mindert-die-Selbstkontrolle.html

22 cf. http://www.nestle.de/themenwelten/einblicke/out-of-home

23 cf. Nestlé Deutschland AG, Studie 2009

24 cf. www/nestle.de/themenwelten/dossier/gluten-und-zoeliakie

25 R. Keller: Klinische Symptomatik "Zöliakie, ein Eisberg". In: Monats-
    schrift Kinderheilkunde. Heidelberg 151.2003, pp. 706–714

26 cf. http://www.nahrungsmittel-intoleranz.com/laktoseintoleranz-infor
    mationen-symptome/ethnische-betrachtung-laktoseintoleranz.html

27 cf. 3sat.online: Laktoseintoleranz ist der Ur-Zustand, broadcast on
    9.10.2014 "Der Feind in meinem Bauch"

28 cf. Gehirn und Geist Nr. 4/2014, p. 76ff

29 Conversation with Stephan Palzer

30 cf. Gehirn und Geist 4/2014

31 cf. EPFL, http://actu.epfl.ch/news/nestle-research-center-and-epfl-unco
    ver-the-medi-2/

32 cf. Nestlé Deutschland AG, Gesund genießen

33 cf. ibid.

34 cf. http://www.nestle.de/themenwelten/dossier/die-ersten-1000-tage

35 cf. Nestlé Lagebericht 2015

36 cf. http://www.nestle.de/themenwelten/news-storys/kochen-mit-kin
    dern

37 cf. Nestlé in der Gesellschaft. Gemeinsame Wertschöpfung und unsere
    sozialen Verpflichtungen 2015

38   cf. http://www.alimentarium.ch/de/academy

39   cf. Shepherd http://www.ncbi.nlm.nih.gov/pmc/articles/PMC406401/

40   cf. http://www.ealimentarium.ch/de/magazine/eine-welt-fuenf-sinne
      Essen mit Sinn und Verstand

41   cf. Thaler

Chapter 8:
Milestones on the way to the future

1   cf. Kussmann/Van Bladeren 2011

2   cf. http://www.nestle.de/themenwelten/einblicke/entstehung-der-zu
     kunftsstudie und http://www.nestle.de/zukunftsstudie

3   cf. http://www.stern.de/wirtschaft/superfoods—acai-beeren—chia-sa
     men-und-goji-beeren-sind-gar-nicht-so-super-6424094.html

4   cf. Der Spiegel Nr. 36/29.8.2015

5   cf. ibid.

6   cf. Frankfurter Allgemeine Zeitung, 7. June 2011

7   cf. Frankfurter Allgemeine Zeitung, 27. January 2015

8   cf. Guriin/Smeaton

LITERATURE

Adler, A. J., Taylor, F., Martin, N., Gottlieb, S., Taylor, R. S., & Ebrahim, S. (2014): Reduced dietary salt for the prevention of cardiovascular disease. The Cochrane Library.

Ahmed, Farooq, Tales of adversity, in: Nature, Vol. 468, 23/30 December 2010

Alexander, E. Y. (2011): Major multinational food and beverage companies and informal sector contributions to global food consumption: implications for nutrition policy. Globalization and health, 7(1), 26.

Ames BN, Elson-Schwab I, Silver EA.: High does vitamin therapy stimulates variant enzymes with decreased coenzyme binding affinity (increased Km): relevance to genetic disease and polymorphisms. AJCN 75, 616 – 658 (2002)

Andlauer, W., & Fürst, P. (2002): Nutraceuticals: a piece of history, present status and outlook. Food Research International, 35(2), 171–176.

Annan, K. & Dryden S. (2016) Food and the Transformation of Africa. Getting Smallholders Connected. The Fourth Industrial Revolution, A Davos Reader, by Gideon Rose.

Astarita, G., & Langridge, J. (2013): An Emerging Role for Metabolomics in Nutrition Science. Journal of nutrigenetics and nutrigenomics, 6(4–5), 179–198.

Astley, S. B., & Elliott, R. M. (2004): The European Nutrigenomics Organisation–linking genomics, nutrition and health research. Nutrition Bulletin, 29(3), 254–261.

Bakker, M. (2014, June 10): Google Food Team's Big Vision for Hacking A Better Future of Dining. (F. T. Connect, Intervieweur)

Ballke, C., & Meisterernst, A. (2012): Nutrigenomics – A new trend from a legal perspective. European Food and Feed Law Review : EFFL, 7(1), 14–21.

Barclay, D./Haschke, F.: The food industry and consumer nutrition and health (2015), World Review of Nutrition and Dietetics, 111, pp. 198–204

Barker DJP, Gluckman PD, Godfrey KM, Harding JE, Owens JA, Robinson JS: Fetal nutrition and cardiovascular disease in adult life. The Lancet 341, 938 (1993)

Beddington, J. (2009). Food, energy, water and the climate: a perfect storm of global events? World Development, 1–9. doi:10.1016/j.funeco.2014.08.001

Belasco, Warren J.: Appetite for Change: How the Counter Culture Took on the Food Industry, 1966–1988, New York 1989

Bergmann, Karin: Industriell gefertigte Lebensmittel. Hoher Wert und schlechtes Image? Berlin 1999

Bergmann, M. M., & Mathers, J. C. (2011): Ethical challenges in human nutrigenomics research. Maturitas, 68(4), 297–298.

Berner, Louise A./Keast, Debra R./Bailey, Regan L./ Dwyer, Johanna T.: Fortified Foods Are Major Contributors to Nutrient Intakes in Diets of US Children and Adolescents, Journal of the Academy of Nutrition and Dietetics, Volume 114, Issue 7, July 2014, Pages 1009–1022

Betoret, E., Betoret, N., Vidal, D., Fito, P. (2011): Functional foods development: Trends and technologies. Trends in Food Science & Technology, 22 (11), 498–508.

Bhardwaj M (2007): From farm to pharma: public health challenges of nutrigenomics. Personalized Med 4: 423–430

Biesalski, Hans Konrad u.a.: Taschenatlas Ernährung, 2015

Bigliardi, B., & Galati, F. (2013). Innovation trends in the food industry: the case of functional foods. Trends in Food Science & Technology, 31(2), 118–129.

Borius-Gunning, A. A. (2014): European Consumer. Healthy Trend for the Food & Beverage Sector. Morgan Stanley Research Europe.

Bouwman, L. I., & van Woerkum, C. (2009). Placing healthy eating in the everyday context: towards an action approach of gene-based personalized nutrition advice. Nutrition and Genomics: Issues of Ethics, Law, Regulation and Communication, 123.

Boyle, M., & Holben, D. (2012). Community Nutrition in Action: An Entrepreneurial Approach. Belmont, CA: Cengage Learning.

Briesen, Detlef: Das gesunde Leben. Ernährung und Gesundheit seit dem 18. Jahrhundert. Frankfurt/New York 2010

Brown, L./van der Ouderaa, F.: Nutritional genomics. Food industry applications from farm to fork (2007) British Journal of Nutrition, 97 (6), pp. 1027–1035

Brownell, K. D./Warner, K. E. (2009): The Perils of Ignoring History: Big Tobacco Played Dirty and Millions Died. How Similar Is Big Food? Milbank Quarterly, 87: 259–294

Bund für Lebensmittelrecht und Lebensmittelkunde e.V. (BLL), Unsere Lebensmittelwirtschaft – eine starke Kraft für Deutschland

Bundesministerium für Bildung und Forschung: Ernährungsforschung. Gesünder essen mit funktionellen Lebensmitteln. Berlin 2010

Id.: Stoffwechselforschung. Wie Ernährung und Gene auf die Gesundheit wirken. Bonn, Berlin 2008

Bundesvereinigung der Deutschen Ernährungsindustrie (BVE): Ernährungsindustrie 2014

Id.: Ernährungsindustrie 2015

Id.: Jahresbericht 2014–2015

Id.: Die Ernährungsindustrie in Zahlen 2015

Buttriss, J.L.: Food reformulation. The challenges to the food industry (2013) Proceedings of the Nutrition Society, 72 (1), pp. 61–69

Carstensen, L.: The New Age of Much Older Age. Time Magazine Feb 12, 2015

Castle, D. (2009): The Personal and the Public in Nutrigenomics. Nutrition and Genomics: issues of ethics, law, regulation and communication (D. Castle and NL Ries, Eds.) pp. 245–262.

Castle, D., Cline, C., Daar, A. S., Tsamis, C., & Singer, P. A. (2006): Nutrients and norms: ethical issues in nutritional genomics. Discovering the Path to Personalized Nutrition, 419–434.

Id.: P. A. Nutritional Genomics: Opportunities and Challenges. Science, Society, and the Supermarket: The Opportunities and Challenges of Nutrigenomics, 1–17.

Caulfield, T., Shelley, J., Bubela, T., & Minaker, L. (2009): Framing nutrigenomics for individual and public health: public representations of an emerging field. Nutrition and genomics: Issues of ethics, law, regulation and communication, 223.

Charisius, Hanno/Friebe, Richard: Bund fürs Leben. Warum Bakterien unsere Freunde sind. Munich 2014

Chou, C. J./Affolter, M. & Kussmann, M. (2011) : A nutrigenomics view of protein intake. macronutrient, bioactive peptides, and protein turnover. Progress in molecular biology and translational science, 108, 51–74

CIAA. (2005). Food and Drink Industry, Initiatives on Diet, Physical Activity and Health. CIAA CONGRESS 2004: Food Futures. Eating Well, Feeling Good. Confederation of the food and drink industries of the EU.

Compher, C., & Mehta, N. M. (2016). Diagnosing Malnutrition: Where Are We and Where Do We Need to Go? *Journal of the Academy of Nutrition and Dietetics,* 116(5), 779–784. doi:10.1016/j.jand.2016.02.001

Confederation of the food and drink industries of the EU CIAA, Data & trends of the European Food and Drink Industry 2009

Constantin, Nathalie/Wahli, Walter: Die Nutrigenomik oder der Köningsweg zu einer präventiven Ernährung, in SVDE (Schweizerischer Verband diplomierter Ernährungsberater/innen) ASDD Info 6/2013

Cordain, L., Eaton, S. B., Sebastian, A., Mann, N., Lindeberg, S., Watkins, B. A., ... & Brand-Miller, J. (2005): Origins and evolution of the Western diet: health implications for the 21st century. The American journal of clinical nutrition, 81(2), 341–354.

Crogan, N. L., & Pasvogel, A. (2003): The influence of protein-calorie malnutrition on quality of life in nursing homes. The Journals of Gerontology Series A: Biological Sciences and Medical Sciences, 58(2), M159-M164.

Darnton-Hill, I., Margetts, B., & Deckelbaum, R. (2004): Public health nutrition and genetics: implications for nutrition policy and promotion. Proceedings of the Nutrition Society, 63(01), 173–185.

DeBusk, R. (2009): Diet-related disease, nutritional genomics, and food and nutrition professionals. Journal of the American dietetic association, 109(3), 410–413.

DeBusk, R. M., Fogarty, C. P., Ordovas, J. M., & Kornman, K. S. (2005): Nutritional genomics in practice: Where do we begin?. Journal of the American dietetic association, 105(4), 589–598.

DeFelice, S. L. (1995). The nutraceutical revolution: its impact on food industry R&D. Trends in Food Science & Technology, 6(2), 59–61.

DeFroidmont-Görtz, I. B. (2009). Emerging technologies and perspectives for nutrition research in European Union 7th Framework Programme. European journal of nutrition, 48(1), 49–51.

Denkwerk Zukunft: Stiftung kulturelle Erneuerung. Factbook 1: Die gegenwärtige und künftige Bedeutung von Essen und Trinken für den gesellschaftlichen Zusammenhalt in Deutschland. Im Auftrag des Zukunftsforums der Nestlé Deutschland AG, Bonn 2010

Dennis, C. A. (2009). Technologies Shaping the Future. Dans FAO, & A. C. da Silva (Ed.), Agro-industries for Development (pp. 92–135). Bodmin: MPG Books Group.

Diabetes Prevention Program Research Group. (2002). Reduction in the incidence of type II diabetes

Der Spiegel Nr. 36/29.8.2015, p. 114 f, Abschied vom Analogkäse

Der Spiegel Wissen 4/2013, Bauchsache p. 108 ff

De Schutter, O. (2014). Report of the Special Rapporteur on the right to food. *Final report: The transformative potential of the right to food.* doi:10.1093/oxfordhb/9780199560103.003.0005.

Deutscher Bauernverband: Situationsbericht 2014/15

Doell, D./Folmer, D./Lee, H./Honigfort, M. & Carberry, S.: Updated estimate of trans fat intake by the US population, Food Additives & Contaminants: Part A Volume 29, Issue 6, 2012

Dwyer, JT, Fulgoni, VL, et al. (2012). Is »Processed« a Four-Letter Word ? The Role of Processed Foods in Achieving Dietary Guidelines. *Adv Nutr*, 3(1), 536–548. doi:10.3945/an.111.000901.536

Earle, M. D. (1997): Innovation in the food industry. Trends in Food Science & Technology, 8(5), 166–175.

European Commission: From farm to fork, Safe food for Europe's consumers, Brüssel 2004.

Ders.: 50 years of Food Safety in the European Union, Luxemburg: Office für Official Publications of the European Communities, 2007

Fallaize, R., Macready, A. L., Butler, L. T., Ellis, J. A., & Lovegrove, J. A. (2013): An insight into the public acceptance of nutrigenomic-based personalised nutrition. Nutrition Research Reviews, 26(1), 39–48. doi:http://dx.doi.org/10.1017/S0954422413000024

Feldman, Z., Bradley, D.G., Greenberg, D. The food and beverage industry's efforts regarding obesity prevention (2010) Obesity Epidemiology: From Aetiology to Public Health

Feng J He, Sonia Pombo-Rodrigues, Graham A MacGregor: Salt reduction in England from 2003 to 2011: its relationship to blood pressure, stroke and ischaemic heart disease mortality BMJ Open 2014;4:e004549

Focus Nr. 30/2013, Wo die Gesundheit sitzt, p. 79 ff.

FoodDrinkEurope: Data & Trends of the European Food and Drink Industry 2013–2014

Frankfurter Allgemeine Zeitung, 7. Juni 2011, Jedermanns Gentest

Frankfurter Allgemeine Zeitung, 25. Oktober 2014, Die Welt ist dem Silicon Valley nicht genug

Frankfurter Allgemeine Zeitung, 27. Januar 2015, Die Fitness-Falle

Fraunhofer-Institut für Verfahrenstechnik und Verpackung (IVV) und Technische Universität München Wissenschaftszentrum Weihenstephan (WZW) Lehrstuhl für Ernährungsphysiologie im Auftrag des deutschen Bundesministeriums für Bildung und Forschung (BMBF) (Ed.): Studie zum Innovationssektor Lebensmittel und Ernährung, Freising/Berlin 2010

Freedhoff, Yoni, and Paul C. Hébert: Partnerships between health organizations and the food industry risk derailing public health nutrition. Canadian Medical Association Journal 183.3 (2011): 291–292.

Fuchs, Richard: Functional Food. Medikamente in Lebensmitteln. Chancen und Risiken. Berlin 1999

Galesi, D. (2014): Towards the Genomization of Food? Potentials and Risks of Nutrigenomics as a Way of Personalized Care and Prevention. Italian Sociological Review, 4(2).

Gedrich, Kurt /Oltersdorf, Ulrich (Eds.): Ernährung und Raum: Regionale und ethnische Ernährungsweisen in Deutschland, Karlsruhe, 2002.

Gehirn und Geist Nr. 4/2014, p. 76ff

GEO kompakt Nr. 42, 2015, p. 30, Wie Essen unser Fühlen bestimmt

German, J. B., Zivkovic, A. M., Dallas, D. C., & Smilowitz, J. T. (2011): Nutrigenomics and personalized diets: what will they mean for food?. Annual review of food science and technology, 2, p. 97–123

Ghosh, D., Skinner, M. A., & Laing, W. A. (2007): Pharmacogenomics and nutrigenomics: Synergies and differences. European Journal of Clinical Nutrition, 61(5), 567–74. doi:http://dx.doi.org/10.1038/sj.ejcn.1602590

Gill, R. (2009): Business applications of nutrigenomics: an industry perspective. Nutrition and genomics. Issues of ethics, laws, regulations and communication, 1st edn. Academic Press/Elsevier, 45–61.

Godard, B., & Ozdemir, V. (2008): Nutrigenomics and personalized diet: from molecule to intervention and nutri-ethics. OMICS: A Journal of Integrative Biology, 12(4), 227+.

Gottlicher M, Widmark E, Li Q, and Gustafsson J-A.: Fatty acids activate a chimera of the clofibric acid-activated receptor and the glucocorticoid receptor. PNAS 89 4653 – 4657 (1993)

Green, H.: Global obesity. Nestlé initiatives in nutrition, health, and wellness (2006), Nutrition Reviews, 64 (SUPPL. 1), pp. S62-S64

Griffin, J. D., & Lichtenstein, A. H. (2013): Dietary cholesterol and plasma lipoprotein profiles: randomized controlled trials. Current nutrition reports, 2(4), 274–282.

Gurrin, Cathal/Smeaton, Alan F./Doherty, Aiden R.: LifeLogging: Personal Big Data, in: Foundations and Trends in Information Retrieval. Vol. 8, No. 1 (2014) 1–107

Harcombe, Z., Baker, J. S., Cooper, S. M., Davies, B., Sculthorpe, N., DiNicolantonio, J. J., & Grace, F. (2015): Evidence from randomised controlled trials did not support the introduction of dietary fat guidelines in 1977 and 1983: a systematic review and meta-analysis. Open heart, 2(1), e000196.

Hawkes, Corinna/Harris, Jennifer L.: An analysis of the content of food industry pledges on marketing to children, Public Health Nutrition 14.08 (2011): 1403–1414.

Heimann, Jim: Car Hops and Curb service. A History of American Drive-In Restaurants 1920–1960. Chronicle Books / Edition Stemmle, Kilchberg 1996.

Hesketh, J.: Personalised nutrition. How far has nutrigenomics progressed? (2013), European Journal of Clinical Nutrition, 67 (5), pp. 430–435.

Hirschfelder, Gunther: Europäische Esskultur: Eine Geschichte der Ernährung von der Steinzeit bis heute, Frankfurt, 2005.

Horrigan, L. L. (2002): How Sustainable Agriculture Can Address the Environmental and Human Health Harms of Industrial Agriculture. Environmental health perspectives, 110(5), 445–456.

Huber M./Knottnerus J. A./Green L./Horst HVD/Jadad AR/ Kromhout D/Leonard B/Lorig K/Loureiro MI/Meet KWMVD/ Schnabel P/Smith R/Weel CV/Smid H.: How should we define health? BMJ 343, d4163-d4163

IDF: Faktenblatt des Internationalen Milchwirtschaftsverbandes Februar 2013

IFIC Foundation. (2009). 2009 Food & Health Survey. Washington, D.C.: International Food Information Council (IFIC) Foundation.

Index, A. t. (2013). Access to Nutrition Index Global Index 2013. Global Alliance for Improved Nutrition.

International Diabetes Federation (IDF): IDF Diabetes Atlas 2014

International Food & Beverage Alliance 2012 Progress Report

Jutzi, Sebastian: Der bewohnte Mensch. Darm, Haut, Psyche. Besser leben mit Mikroben, Munich 2014

Kahlert, Christian/ Müller, Pascal, Mikrobiom – die Entdeckung eines Organs, in: Schweizer Med Forum 2014;14 (16–17):342–344

Kaput, J. (2006): An introduction and overview of nutritional genomics: application to Type 2 diabetes and international nutrigenomics. Nutritional Genomics: Discovering the Path to Personalized Nutrition, 1–35.

Id.: Nutrigenomics research for personalized nutrition and medicine (2008) Current Opinion in Biotechnology, 19 (2), pp. 110–120.

Kaput J, Kussmann M, Mendoza Y, LeCoutre R, Cooper K, Roulin A. Enabling nutrient security and sustainability through systems research. Genes&Nutrition, in press 2015

Kaput J/Morine MJ: Discovery-based nutritional systems biology: developing N-of-1 nutrigenomic research. Int. J for Vitamin and Nutrition Research. 82, 333 -341 (2012)

Kaput J, Ning B. Nutrigenomics for Pet Nutrition and Medicine. Compendum: Continuing Education for Veterinarians. Supplement 31, 40 – 45 (2009)

Kaput, J., Ordovas, J. M., Ferguson, L., Van Ommen, B., Rodriguez, R. L., Allen, L., ... & Korf, B. R. (2005): The case for strategic international alliances to harness nutritional genomics for public and personal health. British Journal of Nutrition, 94(05), 623–632.

Kaput J./ Rodriguez RL.: Nutritional genomics: the next frontier in the post genomic era. Physiological Genomics 16, 166–177. 2004

Ead.: Nutritional Genomics, Discovering the Path to Personalized Nutrition. Wiley and Sons. 2006

Kaput J./Swartz, Paisely E, Mangian H, Daniel WL, Visek WJ: Diet-disease interactions at the molecular level: an experimental paradigm. J. Nutrition 124, 1265S – 1305S

Kauwell, G. (2008). Epigenetics: what it is and how it can affect dietetics practice. Journal of the American Dietetic Association, 108(6), 1056–1059.

Kessler, David: Das Ende des großen Fressens. Wie die Nahrungsmittelindustrie Sie zu übermäßigem Essen verleitet. Was Sie dagegen tun können. Munich 2011

Kilcast, David, and Fiona Angus, eds.: Reducing salt in foods: Practical strategies. Elsevier, 2007.

Klugger, J.: How your Mindset Can Change How You Age. Time Magazine Feb 12, 2015

König, Wolfgang: Geschichte der Konsumgesellschaft (Vierteljahresschrift für Sozial- und Wirtschaftsgeschichte – Beihefte) gebundene Ausgabe 2000

Korthals, M. (2011): Deliberations on the Life Sciences: Pitfalls, Challenges and Solutions. Journal of Public Deliberation, 7(1), 8.

Korthals, M., & Komduur, R. (2010): Uncertainties of nutrigenomics and their ethical meaning. Journal of Agricultural and Environmental Ethics, 23(5), 435–454. doi:http://dx.doi.org/10.1007/s10806-009-9223-0

Korver, O.:›Healthy‹ developments in the food industry (1997) Cancer Letters, 114 (1–2), pp. 19–23

Kris-Etherton, P.M., Lefevre, M., R.P. Mensink, et al: »Trans Fatty Acid Intakes and Food Sources in the U.S. Population: NHANES 1999–2002«, Lipids October 2012, Volume 47, Number 10, pp. 931–940

Krul, E. S., & Gillies, P. J. (2009): Translating nutrigenomics research into practice: the example of soy protein. Nutrition and Genomics: Issues of Ethics, Law, Regulation and Communication, 25.

Kussmann, M., & Van Bladeren, P. J. (2011). The extended nutrigenomics – understanding the interplay between the genomes of food, gut microbes, and human host, in:. Frontiers in genetics 2. 2011, Vol. 2, Article 21

Kussmann, M., Blum, S. (2007): OMICS-derived targets for inflammatory gut disorders: opportunities for the development of nutrition related biomarkers. Endocrine, Metabolic & Immune Disorders-Drug Targets (Formerly Current Drug Targets-Immune, Endocrine & Metabolic Disorders), 7(4), 271–287

Kussmann, Martin/Fay, Laurent B.: Nutrigenomics and personalized nutrition: Science and concept (2008) in: Personalized Medicine, 5 (5), pp. 447–455.

Kussmann, Hager, Morine, Kaput: Systems Diabetes Frontiers 2013, 4, 205

Kussmann, M./Rezzi, S./Daniel, H. (2008): Profiling techniques in nutrition and health research. Current opinion in biotechnology, 19(2), 83–99.

Kussmann/Siffert: NutritionEpiGenetics, NutrRev 2010, 68, pp. 38–47

Lang, Timothy/Heasman, Michael: Food wars: the global battle for minds, mouths, and markets, Sterling/USA 2004

Larson IA, Ordovas JM, Barnard JR, Hoffmann MM, Feussner G, Lamon-Fava S, Schaefer EJ: Effects of apolipoprotein A-I genetic variations on plasma apolipoprotein, serum lipoprotein and glucose levels. Clin Genet 61, 176 – 184. (2002).

Laursen, L. (2010): Interdisciplinary research: Big science at the table. Nature, 468 (7327), pp. 2–4.

Leitzmann, Claus/Cannon, Geoffrey: Die Gießener Erklärung zum Projekt »Die neue Ernährungswissenschaft«, in: Ernährungs-Umschau 53 (2006) Heft 2

Leitzmann, Claus et al.: Ernährung in Prävention und Therapie: Ein Lehrbuch, 2009

Ludwig, D.S./Nestle, M.: Can the food industry play a constructive role in the obesity epidemic? (2008) JAMA – Journal of the American Medical Association, 300 (15), pp. 1808–1811

Maddison, Angus: The World Economy – A Millenial Perspective, Paris 2001

Menzel, Peter/D'Alusio, Faith: What the World Eats, 2008

Metro AG (Ed.): Metro-Handelslexikon 2014/2015, Düsseldorf, 2014

Mine, Y., Miyashita, K., & Shahidi, F. (2009): Nutrigenomics and proteomics in health and disease: An overview. Nutrigenomics and Proteomics in Health and Disease: Food Factors and Gene Interactions, 1.

Moco, S., Candela, M., Chuang, E., Draper, C., Cominetti, O., Montoliu, I., ... & Martin, F. P. J. (2014): Systems Biology Approaches for Inflammatory Bowel Disease: Emphasis on Gut Microbial Metabolism. Inflammatory bowel diseases, 20(11), 2104–2114.

Montoliu, I./Scherer, M./Beguelin, F./DaSilva, L./Mari, D./ Salvioli, S., ... & Collino, S. (2014): Serum profiling of healthy aging identifies phospho-and sphingolipid species as markers of human longevity. Aging (Albany NY), 6(1), 9.

Morine, M. J., Monteiro, J. P., Wise, C., Pence, L., Williams, A., Ning, B., McCabe-Sellers, B., Champagne, C., Turner, J., Shelby, B., Bogle, M., Beger, R. D., Priami, C.: Genetic associations with micronutrient levels identified in immune and gastrointestinal networks. Genes&Nutrition

Moss, Mchael: Salt Sugar Fat. How the Food Giants Hooked Us. New York 2013

Id., Das Salz Zucker Fett Komplott. Wie die Lebensmittelkonzerne uns süchtig machen, Munich, 2014

Naisbitt, John: Megatrends. 10 Perspektiven, die unser Leben verändern werden, Munich, 1985

Nestlé AG (Hrsg.): Heer, Jean: Nestlé hundertfünfundzwanzig Jahre von 1866 bis 1991, Vevey 1991

Id.: Nestlé Research and Development at the dawn of the 21st Century, 2000

Id.: People building brands, 2000

Id.: The World Food Company, 2001

Id.: (Ed.) Pfiffner, Albert/Renk, Hans-Jörg: Wandel als Herausforderung. Nestlé 1990–2005, Cham und Vevey 2007

Id.: Innovating the future. Research & Development for Nutrition, Health and Wellness, 2007

Id.: Ernährungsbedürfnisse und hochwertige Ernährung, Bericht zur Gemeinsamen Wertschöpfung 2008

Id.: Nestlé Good Food Good Life Trends. Understanding trends in nutrition, health and wellness. Wellness in action. fast forward to Good Food, Good Life. 2011, July

Id.: Nestlé in society – Creating Shared Value and meeting our commitments, 2014

Id.: Nestlé in der Gesellschaft, Gemeinsame Wertschöpfung und unsere sozialen Verpflichtungen, 2014

Id.: Annual Report 2014

Id.: Corporate Governance Report 2014, Compensation Report 2014, Financial Statements 2014

Id.: Jahresbericht 2014

Id.: Henri Nestlé 1814–1890. From Pharmacist's Assistant to Founder of the World's Leading Nutrition, Health and Wellness Company. Cham/Vevey 2014

Id: Nestlé Policy on Micronutrient Fortification of Foods & Beverages, Poliy Mandatory, June 2015

Nestlé Deutschland AG: Nestlé Studie 2009. Ernährung in Deutschland 2008

Id.: Nestlé Studie 2011. So is(s)t Deutschland. Ein Spiegel der Gesellschaft

Id.: Nestlé Studie 2012. Das is(s)t Qualität

Ders.: Gesund genießen. Essen und Trinken für mehr Wohlbefinden

Id.: Bericht zur gemeinsamen Wertschöpfung 2014. Qualität nehmen wir wörtlich

Nestlé Fondation Alimentarium: Gen-Welten Ernährung

Nestle, Marion: Food politics: How the food industry influences nutrition and health.

Nestlé Research: Vision, Action, Value Creation, 2010

Nestlé Research Center: The Fountain of Knowledge. Research for Nutrition, Health and Wellness, 2004

Nestlé Zukunftsforum/tns infratest: NZF-Factbook II, Consumer Confusion

Neue Zürcher Zeitung Publishing: Business in a Changing Society. Festschrift für Peter Brabeck-Letmathe, Zürich 2014

Oaklander, M: How to Live Longer. Time Magazine Feb 12, 2015

Offord, E., Major, G., Vidal, K., Gentile-Rapinett, G., Baetge, E., Beck, T., & le Coutre, J.: Nutrition throughout life: innovation for healthy ageing.

van Ommen, B., Keijer, J., Heil, S. G., Kaput, J.: Challenging homeostasis to define biomarkers for nutrition related health. Molecular Nutrition Food Research 53, 795– 804 (^{2}2009)

Ordovas, J., & Shyong Tai, E. (2009): Gene–Environment Interactions: Where are we and where should we be Going?. Nutrition and Genomics: Issues of Ethics, Law, Regulation and Communication, 1.

Ornish, D.:. It's Time to Embrace Lifestyle Medicine. Time Magazine Feb 12, 2015

Pan, Y. (2011): Enhancing brain functions in senior dogs: a new nutritional approach. Topics in companion animal medicine, 26(1), 10–16.

Id.: Cognitive dysfunction syndrome in dogs and cats. CAB Reviews 2013 8, No. 051 (2013)

Id.: Enhancing cognitive function through diet in cats. Nestle Purina Companion Animal Nutrition Summit: Nutrition for Life. March 27–29, 2014, Austin, Texas

Pan, Y., Larson, B., Araujo, J. A., Lau, W., De Rivera, C., Santana, R., ... & Milgram, N. W. (2010): Dietary supplementation with medium-chain TAG has long-lasting cognition-enhancing effects in aged dogs. British journal of nutrition, 103(12), 1746–1754

Panchaud, A., Affolter, M., & Kussmann, M. (2012): Mass spectrometry for nutritional peptidomics: how to analyze food bioactives and their health effects. Journal of proteomics, 75(12), 3546–3559

Park, A.: The Cure for Aging. Time Magazine Feb 12, 2015

Park, E., Paisely, E., Mangian, H.J., Swartz, D.A., Wu, M.X., O'Morchoe, P.J., Behr, S.R., visek WJ, Kaput, J.: Lipid level and type alter stearoyl CoA desaturase mRNA abundance differently in mice with distinct susceptibilities to diet-influenced diseases. J Nutrition 127

Pendergrast, Mark: Für Gott und Coca-Cola. Die unautorisierte Geschichte der Coca-Cola Company. Munich, 1993

Id.: Uncommon Grounds. The History of Coffee and How It Transformed Our World. 1999

Penders, B., Horstman, K., Saris, W. H., & Vos, R. (2007): From individuals to groups: a review of the meaning of ›personalized‹in nutrigenomics.

Perlmutter, David: Brain Maker. The Power of Gut Microbes to Heal and Protect Your Brain – for Life, 2015

Peters, Achim: Das egoistische Gehirn. Warum unser Kopf Diäten sabotiert und gegen den eigenen Körper kämpft, Berlin, 2008

Pollan, Michael: 64 Grundregeln Essen. Essen Sie nichts, was Ihre Großmutter nicht als Essen erkannt hätte. Munich, 2011

Qi, L.: Personalized nutrition and obesity (2014), Annals of Medicine, 46 (5), pp. 247–252

Reed, M.N., Doll, D., Simpkins, J.W., & Barr, T. (2014): Aging & stroke: The human condition. Proceedings Nestle Purina Companion Animal Nutrition Summit: Nutrition for Life. March 27–29, 2014, Austin, Texas.

Reilly, P. R., & DeBusk, R. M. (2008): Ethical and legal issues in nutritional genomics. Journal of the American dietetic association, 108(1), 36–40.

Rockhill B, Newman C, Wienberg R.: Use and misuse of population attributable fractions. Am Journal Public Health. 88, 15 – 19. (1998)

Ronald, P.C. & Adamchak R.W. (2008) Tomorrow's Table : Organic Farming, Genetics and the Future of Food. Oxford University Press.

Ronteltap, A., van Trijp, J. C. M., & Renes, R. J. (2007): Expert views on critical success and failure factors for nutrigenomics. Trends in food science & technology, 18(4), 189–200.

Ead.: (2008): Making nutrigenomics work–Integrating expert stakeholder opinions and consumer preferences. Trends in food science & technology, 19(7), 390–398. Trends in food

science & technology, 18(6), 333–338.

Saguy, Sam I. (2011): Paradigm shifts in academia and the food industry required to meet innovation challenges. Trends in Food Science & Technology, 22(9), 467–475.

Schwarz, Friedhelm: Nestlé. Macht durch Nahrung. Munich, 2000

Id.: Nestlé. The Secrets of Food, Trust and Globalization, Toronto, 2002

Id.: Nestlé. Macht durch Nahrung, Bergisch Gladbach 2003

Scriver, C.: Nutrient-gene interactions. The gene is not the disease and vice versa

Sela, D. C. (2008): The genome sequence of Bifidobacterium longum subsp. infantis reveals adaptations for milk utilization within the infant microbiome. Proceedings of the National Academy of Sciences, 105(48), 18964–69.

Sifferlin, A.: What Diet Helps People Live the Longest? Time Magazine. Feb 12, 2015.

Simopoulos, A. P., Bourne, P. G., & Faergeman, O. (2013): Bellagio report on healthy agriculture, healthy nutrition, healthy people. Nutrients, 5(2), 411–423. doi:http://dx.doi.org/10.3390/nu5020411

Sloan, E. (2002): The top 10 functional food trends: the next generation. Food Technologies, 56(4), 32–57.

Spiekermann, Uwe: Nahrung und Ernährung im Industriezeitalter, in: Materialien zur Ermittlung von Ernährungsverhalten, 35 – 73, Karlsruhe, 1997.

Id.: Basis der Konsumgesellschaft: Entstehung und Entwicklung des modernen Kleinhandels in Deutschland 1850–1914 (Schriftenreihe zur Zeitschrift für Unternehmensgeschichte) 1999

Stauffer, J. E. (2004): Nutrigenomics. Cereal Foods World, 49(4), 247–248. Retrieved from http://search.proquest.com/docview/230356946?accountid=13876

Stover, P. J., & Caudill, M. A. (2008): Genetic and epigenetic contributions to human nutrition and health: managing genome–diet interactions. Journal of the American Dietetic Association, 108(9), 1480–1487.

Subbiah, M. R. (2008): Understanding the nutrigenomic definitions and concepts at the food-genome junction. OMICS A Journal of Integrative Biology, 12(4), 229–235.

Talbot, G.: Reducing Saturated Fats in Foods 2011 Woodhead Publishing Limited

Technoseum Landesmuseum für Technik und Arbeit in Mannheim (Ed.): Unser täglich Brot ... Die Industrialisierung der Ernährung: Katalog zur Ausstellung vom 28.10.2011–29.4.2012, Mannheim, 2011.

Teicholz, Nina: The Big Fat Surprise: Why Butter, Meat and Cheese belong in a Healthy Diet, 2014

Teuteberg, Hans J./Wiegelmann, Günter: Nahrungsgewohnheiten in der Industrialisierung des 19. Jahrhunderts, Berlin, 2005

Thaler, Richard H./Sunstein, Cass R.: Nudge. Improving Decisions About Health, Whealth, and Happiness, 2008

The Lancet 2014: Contribution of six risk factors to achieving the 25×25 non-communicable disease mortality reduction target: a modelling study Kontis, Vasilis et al. The Lancet, Volume 384, Issue 9941, 427 – 437

The Nielsen Company. (2014). Snack Attack. What Consumers are reaching for Around the World. Nielsen Global Survey of Snacking.

Thomas, D., & Frankenberg, E. (2002): Health, nutrition and prosperity: a microeconomic perspective. Bulletin of the World Health Organization, 80(2), 106–113.

Topol, E. J.: (2012). The creative destruction of medicine: How the digital revolution will create better health care. Basic Books.

Id.: (2014): Individualized medicine from prewomb to tomb. Cell, 157(1), 241–253. http://www.ncbi.nlm.nih.gov /pubmed/24679539

United Nations (UN), 1973, The Determinants and Consequences of Population Trends, Population Studies, No. 50

United Nations Department of Economic and Social Affairs Popular Division: World Population Prospects. The 2015 Revision. Key findings and Advance Tables, New York 2015

USDA: Research Investments and Market Structure in the Food Processing, Agricultural Input, and Biofuel Industries Worldwide, Executive Summary, Economic Information Bulletin Number 90, December 2011, http://www.ers.usda.gov/media/193646/eib90_1_.pdf

Verbraucherzentrale Bundesverband e.V. (vzbv) (Ed.): Essen im Alter, 2004.

Virmani, A., Pinto, L., Binienda, Z., & Ali, S. (2013). Food, Nutrigenomics, and Neurodegeneration—Neuroprotection by What You Eat!. Molecular neurobiology, 48(2), 353–362.

Voûte, J./Heughan, A./Casimiro, J.: Non-communicable diseases and the food and beverage industry (2012) The Lancet, 379 (9814), pp. 410–411

Wanjek, C. (2005): Food at work: Workplace solutions for malnutrition, obesity and chronic diseases. Geneva: International Labour Office.

Warner A. (2016) Processed food bad, natural food good ? We got it so wrong. New Scientist, April 28th, 2016.

Weaver, C.M., Dwyer, J., Fulgoni III, V.L., King, J.C., Leveille, G.A., MacDonald, R.S., Ordovas, J., Schnakenberg, D.: Processed foods. Contributions to nutrition (2014) American Journal of Clinical Nutrition, 99 (6), pp. 1525–1542

Weaver, John D.: Carnation. the first 75 Years 1899–1974, 1974

Webster, J.; Trieu, K.; Dunford, E.; Hawkes, C.: Target Salt 2025: A Global Overview of National Programs to Encourage the Food Industry to Reduce Salt in Foods. Nutrients 2014, 6, 3274–3287

Wen Ng, Shu, Slining, Meghan M., Barry M. Popkin: The Healthy Weight Commitment Foundation Pledge: Calories Sold from U.S. Consumer Packaged Goods, 2007–2012, American Journal of Preventive Medicine, Volume 47, Issue 4, October 2014, Pages 508–519

WHO Global status report of noncommunicable diseases 2014

Williams, R. Biochemical Individuality: The Basis for the Genetotrophic Concept

Wolff GL, Kodell RL, Moore SR, Cooeny CA: Maternal epigenetics and methyl supplements affect agouti gene expression in Avy/a mice. FASEB Journal12, 949 – 957 (1998)

Yach, D.: Food companies and nutrition for better health (2008) Public Health Nutrition, 11 (2), pp. 109–111.

Yach, D., Lucio, A., Barroso, C. Can food and beverage companies help improve population health? Some insights from PepsiCo (2007) Medical Journal of Australia, 187 (11–12), pp. 656–657.

Yach, Derek MBCHC, MPH, Feldman, Zoë MPH, Dondeena Bradley PHD, Robert Brown: Preventive Nutrition and the Food Industry: Perspectives on History, Present, and Future Directions, Preventive Nutrition 2010, pp 769–792

Yach, D., Khan, M., Bradley, D., Hargrove, R., Kehoe, S., Mensah, G.: Young, V. R., & Scrimshaw, N. S. (1979). Genetic and biological variability in human nutrient requirements. The American journal of clinical nutrition, 32(2), 486–500

Zachwieja, J., Hentges, E., Hill, J.O., Black, R., Vassileva, M. Public-private partnerships: The evolving role of industry funding in nutrition research (2013) Advances in Nutrition, 4 (5), pp. 570–572

Zeit Magazin 11/2013.

Zivkovic, A.M., Smilowitz, J.T., Bruce German, J. Nutrigenomics and Personalized Diets: What Will They Mean for Food? (2011) Food Science and Technology, 25 (1), pp. 36–39.

Internet

3sat.online: Laktoseintoleranz ist der Ur-Zustand, Sendung vom 9.10.2014 »Der Feind in meinem Bauch«.

Agency for Science, Technology and Research http://www.a-star.edu.sg/Media/News/Press-Releases/ID/3816/Infant-gut-microbiota-linked-with-gestation-duration-delivery-method-and-healthy-weight-gain.aspx

Alcock, Joe/Maley, Carlo C./Aktipis, C. Athena: Is eating behavior manipulated by the gastrointestinal microbiota? Evolutionary pressures and potential mechanismus, in: Bioessays 36: 940–949, www.bioessays.de

http://www.alimentarium.ch/de/academy

http://www.bauernverband.de/11-wirtschaftliche-bedeutung-des-agrarsektors-638269

BDSI Bundesverband der Deutschen Süßwarenindustrie Eis Info-Service http://www.markeneis.de/datenfakten

http://www.biography.com/people/clarence-birdseye-9213147

Boyle, M. (2014, May 28): Nestle Accelerates Health-Care Shift With $1.4 Billion Buy. Consulté le February 20, 2015, sur Bloomberg: http://www.bloomberg.com/news/articles/2014-05-28/nestle-sheds-galderma-ties-with-1-4-billion-skin-care-plunge

Bruce, B. (2014, December 14): New Nutrition Business' 10 Key Trends in Food, Nutrition and Health 2015. Consulté le February 9, 2015, sur Food & Beverage International: http://www.foodbev.com/news/new-nutrition-business-10-key-trends-in

www.bve-online.de/download/deutsche-ernaerungsindustrie2015

https://www.bve-online.de/download/bve-statistikbroschuere2014

http://www.bve-online.de/themen/verbraucher/industrielle-produktion/wirtschaftliche-bedeutung

http://www.bve-online.de/themen/branche-und-markt/branchenportrait

http://cailler.ch/de/alles-uber-cailler/geschichte/19-jahrhundert/

http://cailler.ch/de/alles-uber-cailler/geschichte/20-jahrhundert/

http://www.campbellsoupcompany.com/about-campbell/

http://www.census.gov/population/projections/data/

CGF. (2013): Health & Wellness. Consulté le February 28, 2015, sur The Consumer Goods Forum: http://www.theconsumergoodsforum.com/images/the_forum_images/resources/multimedia/infographics/Measuring_Health_and_Wellness_Progress_Infographic.png

Denning, S. (2014, October 9): What's the Future of the Food Industry? Consulté le January 13, 2015, sur Forbes: http://www.forbes.com/sites/stevedenning/2014/09/10/whats-the-future-of-the-food-industry/

http://www.diaetologen.at/fileadmin/user_upload/documents/Kongress/Abstracts_Ernaehrungskongress/Holzer.pdf

http://www.ealimentarium.ch/de/magazine/eine-wlt-fuenf-sinne Essen mit Sinn und Verstand

http://earlybirddiabetes.org./findings.php

EPFL: Nestlé Research Center and EPFL uncover the medicinal power of spices, http://actu.epfl.ch/news/nestle-research-center-and-epfl-uncover-the-medi-2/

EpiGen Global Research Consortium, Press Release 4th February 2015 http://www.epigengrc.com/news

European Food Information Council (EUFIC): Food Today. Who's who der internationalen und europäischen Lebensmittelsicherheit und Ernährung? http://www.eufic.org/article/de/artid/who-is-who-internationale-europaeische-lebensmittelsicherheita-ernaehrung/

http://www.fh-erfurt.de/lgf/fileadmin/GB/Dokumente/Forschung/Bioaktive_Substanzen_im_Gemuese.pdf

FoodBev. (2015, February 15): New beauty drink is first to be enriched with fruit skin macroantioxidants. Consulté le February 16, 2015, sur FoodBev: http://www.foodbev.com/ news/new-beauty-drink-is-first-to-be-enriched

FoodBev. (2015, February 27); Sales of organic products rise, despite an overall fall in food spending. Consulté le March 18, 2015, sur FoodBev: http://www.foodbev. com/news/ sales-of-organic-products-rise-despite-a#.VPmFJUvdvHg

https://www.futuremanagementgroup.com/.../Transhumanismus?

http://www.geoba.se/population.php?pc=world&type=15

Goran, Michael I./Luc Tappy, Kim-Anne: Dietary Sugars and Health Lêhttp://www. crcpress.com/product/isbn/9781466593770

Griffin, E. (2014, April 10): Food startups are cookin': Munchery raises $28 million for meal delivery. Consulté le January 29, 2015, sur Fortune: http://fortune.com/ 2014/04/10/food-startups-are-cookin-munchery-raises-28-million-for-me al-delivery/healthon.de

www.heart.org

http://www.heinzketchup.de/UeberHeinz/OurHistory

IBM-WildDucks. (2015): Message from Mars: Big Data and Genomics Can Make Our Food Safer. Consulté le February 3, 2015, sur IBM: http://www.ibm.com/ smarterplanet/us/en/dispatches/wildducks/mars/#pod

IDFA International Dairy Food Association

http://www.idfa.org/news-views/media-kits/ice-cream

Insights, C. (2014, October 30): Corporate Investment into Digital Health & Health IT Industry Hits Record Level. Consulté le February 12, 2015, sur CB Insights: https://www.cbinsights.com/blog/corporate-digital-health-investment-2014/

http://www.kelloggs.de/de_DE/who-we-are-landing/our-history.html

Kussmann, Martin/ Dean, Jennifer/ Middleton P./ van Bladeren, Peter J./le Coutre, Johannes: Harnessing the power of epigenetics for targeted nutrition http://www. research.nestle.com/resources/downloads/Documents/Nestl%C3%A9%20 White%20paper%20Nutrigenomics %20FINAL.pdf

Kussmann, Martin/Krause, Lutz/Siffert, Winfried: Nutrigenomics: where are we with genetic and epigenetic markers for disposition and suspectibility

http://onlinelibrary.wiley.com/doi/10.1111/j.1753-4887.2010.00326.x/abstract

http://www.the-linde-group.com/internet.global.thelindegroup.global/de/images/ chronik_d%5B1%5D16_9855.pdf

Mellentin, J. (2014, November 3): Key Trends in Functional Foods & Beverages for 2015: Understanding and connecting multiple trends can lead to long-term market success. Consulté le February 20, 2015, sur Nutraceuticals World: http://www.nutraceuticalsworld.com/issues/2014-11/view_features/key-trends-in-functional-foods-beverages-for-2015/

Mintel: Snacking Motivations and Attitudes US 2015

http://mintel.com

Nestlé: Nutrition landscaping for effective fortification, Pressemitteilung vom 16. Oktober 2013

http://www.nestle.com/Media/NewsAndFeatures/

http://www.research.nestle.com/newscenter /news/nestl%C3%A9researchcenteran nouncescollaborationwithepigen,aleadingconsortiumforepigeneticsresearch

http://www.nestle.com/media/newsandfeatures/nestle-research-epigenetics

http://www.research.nestle.com/newscenter/news/correct-nutrition-has-cognition-enhancing-benefits-for-older-cats, Cognition-enhancing benefits for older cats

http://www.nestle.com/media/newsandfeatures/nestle-purina-petcare-thermal-imaging-research, Can people make their pets happy?

Nestlé: Unlocking the metabolic ›master switch‹ to potentially echo exercise effect, Press Release Nov 19, 2014 http://www.nestle.com/media/ newsandfeatures/ ampk-metabolic-master-switch

Nestlé: The Nestlé Healthy Kids Global Programme

http://www.nestle.com/nutrition-health-wellness/kids-best-start/childen-family/healthy-kids-programme

http://www.nestle.de/themenwelten/einblicke/out-of-home

www/nestle.de/themenwelten/dossier/gluten-und-zoeliakie

http://www.nestle.de/themenwelten/einblicke/entstehung-der-zukunftsstudie

http://www.nestle.de/themenwelten/news-storys/lebensmittel-solar-impulse, Lebensmittel entwickelt für extreme Situationen

http://www.nestle.de/themenwelten/news-storys/ernaehrung-der-zukunft-stoffwechsel

http://www.nestle.de/themenwelten/dossier/die-ersten-1000-tage

http://www.nestle.de/themenwelten/news-storys/kochen-mit-kindern

http://www.nestle.de/zukunftsstudie

https://www.nestlehealthscience.com/newsroom/press-releases/the-role-of-nutrition-in-dementia-prevention-and-management

https://www.nestlehealthscience.de/Ern%C3%A4hrungsthemen/HCP/Kau-und-Schluckst%C3%B6rung

https://www.nestlehealthscience.com/newsroom/press-releases/the-role-of-nutrition-in-dementia-prevention-and-management

NIHS News from the Institute NIHS 3.5.2015, Nestlé Institute of Health Science steps up a gear in the fight against muscle loss in old age

https://www.nestleinstitutehealthsciences.com/news/newsinstitute/nestl%C3%A9%20institute%20of%20health%20sciences%20steps%20up%20a%20gear%20in%20the%20fight%20against%20muscle%20loss%20in%20old%20age

https://www.nestleinstitutehealthsciences.com/news/newsinstitute/press-release-three

http://www.nestle-marktplatz.de/view/Marken/Libbys

Nestlé Nutrition Institute: The pattern of Infant's gut bacteria: Biomarkers of future food allergy?

https://www.nestlenutrition-institute.org/country/in/News/Pages/the-pattern-of-infants-gut-bacteria-biomarkers-of-future-food-allergy.aspx

http://ourworldindata.org/data/population-growth-vital-statistics/life-expectancy/

Purina: https://www.purinavets.eu/home/feline/innovations/ageing.htm

Neuroscience News. Do Gut Bacteria Rule Our Minds?

Neurociencenews.com

pharmazeutische-zeitung.de Ausgabe 18 aus 2011

http://www.planet-wissen.de/natur/forschung/epigenetik/pwwbepigenetik100.html

Purina: https://www.purinavets.eu/home/feline/innovations/ageing.htm

Pwc Deutschland: http://www.pwc.de/de/handel-und-konsumguter/usa-verschaer fen-regulierung-zur-lebensmittelsicherheit.html

Shapiro, H. (2015, January 13). Science AMA Series. Consulté le January 21, 21, sur The New Reddit Journal of Science: https://www.reddit.com/r/science/ comments/2s9vhk/science_ama_series_im_howardyana_shapiro_chief

Shepherd, Gordon M.: The Human Sense of Smell: Are we better Than We Think? http://www.ncbi.nlm.nih.gov/pmc/articles/PMC406401/

Simpson, Stephen J./ Raubenheimer, David: The Nature of Nutrition (press.prince ton.edu) http://press.princeton.edu/titles/9776.html

Smith, D. P. (2014). Nestlé Reformulates Products to Improve Nutrition. Consulté le February 10, 2015, sur Shared Value Initiative: http://sharedvalue.org/groups nestl%C3%A9-reformulates-products-improve-nutrition

http://www.spektrum.de/lexikon/geographie/ agrobusiness/191

http://www.spiegel.de/gesundheit/diagnose/demenz-zahl-der-erkrankten-steigt-in-zukunft-rasant-a-937318.html

http://www.spiegel.de/gesundheit/ernaehrung/nutrigenomik-und-individuelle-erna ehrung-essen-was-den-genen-schmeckt-a-936842.html

http://de.statista.com/statistik/daten/studie/2995/umfrage/entwicklung-der-weltweiten-mobilfunkteilnehmer-seit-1993

stern.de vom 10.10.2010

http://www.stern.de/wirtschaft/superfoods-acai-beeren-chia-samen-und-goji-beeren-sind-gar-nicht-so-super-6424094.html

http://suite101.de/article/steckruebenwinter-im-ersten-weltkrieg-a62563

http://time.com/3706693/its-time-to-embrace-lifestyle-medicine/

TomorrowFocusMedia,http://www.forward-adgroup.de/fileadmin/customer_files/pub lic_files/downloads/studien/TFM_SocialTrends_Gesundheit.pdf?PHPSES SID=295e1c582953f740d0d9fc8d12bda56c

Transgenerational Design Matters, The Demographics of Aging, http://transgenera tional.org/demographics.html

http://www.un.org/depts/german/millennium/MDG%20Report%202013_german.pdf

UN/ESA: http://esa.un.org/unup

http://esa.un.org/unpd/wup/highlights/wup2014-highlights.pdf

United States Department of Agriculture Economic Research Service http://ers.usda. gov/data-products/ag-and-food-statistics-charting-the-essentials/ag-and-food-sectors-and-the-economy.aspx

U.S. Department of Health & Human Services http://www.cdc.gov/chronicdisease/

Verband forschender Arzneimittelhersteller: http://www.vfa-bio.de/vb-de/aktuelle-themen/forschung/mikrobiom.html

http://www.vulkane.net/vulkanismus/katastrophen/tambora.html

http://www.weck.de/index.php/ueber-uns

WEF. (2015): New Vision for Agriculture, A global initiative of the World Economic Forum. Consulté le January 9, 2015, sur World Economic Forum: http://www3. weforum.org /docs/WEF_CO_NVA_Overview.pdf

http://www.welt.de/gesundheit/psychologie/article144879242/Schon-leichter-Stress-mindert-die-Selbstkontrolle.html

http://www.welt.de/13707602

http://www.welt.de/kultur/history/article106227344/Es-war-ein-Pilz-der-eine-Million-Iren-toetete.html

WHO: Bulletin of the World Health Organization http://www.who.int/bulletin/volumes/93/4/15- 154831/en/, Keiji Fukuda, Food safety in a globalized world

WHO Codex Alimentarus Commission, http://www.who.int/mediacentre/events/meetings/2015/codex-alimentarius-commission/en/

WHO Media centre: Food safety. Fact sheet 399, November 2014 http://www.who.int/mediacentre/factsheets/fs399/en/

http://www.who.int/gho/mortality_burden_disease/life_tables/situation_trends/en/

World Health Summit http://www.worldhealthsummit.org/

http://www.zeit.de/2012/17/Riesenreich-China/seite-4

Zukunftsinstitut https://www.zukunftsinstitut.de

Nestlé CT-ENT Charts Economics and Context ob/tv #4

Nestlé CT-ENT Charts Economics and Context ob/tv #14

ACKNOWLEDGEMENTS

This book describes developments, changes, the emergence of new knowledge and insights, and their implementation in the economy and society. Some of these developments I have influenced over the past decades, within the range of my possibilities. As a result, all of the changes that have taken place have always been for the benefit of the community.

Without countless conversations with professionals within Nestlé, about science and politics, in government and non-governmental organizations and with customers and suppliers, new ideas could hardly have taken shape which have led and continue to lead to concrete solutions.

I therefore thank all those with whom I have talked and discussed, and who made suggestions or formulated expectations and criticism. I thank you for allowing me to listen and that you listened to me. By comparing ideas new impetuses are given, and new images formed of a realistic and better future. To this extent, this book should be a spur to further fruitful dialogue in which the maximum number of people should participate.

INDEX